VEGAN SLOW COOKER

The Vegan Slow Cooker Cookbook - Delicious, Savory Vegan Recipes

(Vegan Diet Recipes That You Cant Live Without)

Robert Knotts

Published by Sharon Lohan

© **Robert Knotts**

All Rights Reserved

Vegan Slow Cooker: The Vegan Slow Cooker Cookbook - Delicious, Savory Vegan Recipes (Vegan Diet Recipes That You Cant Live Without)

ISBN 978-1-990334-33-7

Legal & Disclaimer

The information contained in this book is not designed to replace or take the place of any form of medicine or professional medical advice. The information in this book has been provided for educational and entertainment purposes only.

Table of contents

Part 1

Chapter 1: Slow Cooker Benefits

Ever since their invention in the 1970s, many people have loved slow cookers for the freedom and meal preparation alternatives they provide. Slow cooking meals has since become a popular alternative to actively slaving over the stove for an hour or more at a time. Slow cookers are also a great choice for those who are looking for healthier eating opportunities but don't feel as though they have the time for traditional meal preparation. The slow-cooking action automatically blends disparate flavors together, creating fantastic tastes without all the trial and error related to more traditional cooking methods.

What's more, studies show that cooking food this way actually improve its nutritional value by increasing the bioavailability of nutrients. This is especially true when it comes to tomatoes as heated tomatoes are known to produce more lycopene than their raw counterparts which is an antioxidant related to heart health.

The same also goes for lutein, an antioxidant that promotes eye health that is found in spinach and corn in higher amounts after these ingredients have been cooked using a slow cooker. Legumes respond the best of all to heat, giving off up to four times as many antioxidants after they have been cooked using a slow cooker than they contain when raw.

Foods that are cooked at higher temperatures are also more likely to produce what are known as advanced glycation end products or AGEs. These AGEs are a form of toxin which is easily absorbed into the body during consumption and have been linked to kidney disease, Alzheimer's disease, vascular issues, diabetes, insulin resistance and inflammation. This is where slow cooking especially shines as the low temperatures typically used reduce the risk of AGEs in vegetables entirely.

In addition, using a slow cooker will provide you with the ability to decrease the amount of processed foods that you consume on a regular basis. Starting a meal in the morning and knowing it is waiting for you at the end of the day will make it much easier to avoid grabbing something processed on the way home, and you can even take the leftovers to lunch the next day meaning you don't have to resort to processed foods when it comes to actively remaining vegan.

In order to get the most out of your slow cooker, it is important to consider the differences between it and other types of meal preparation and plan accordingly. Vegetables that are extra firm are a good choice as they will soften up when given the change.

It is also important to consider how to season slow cooker meals properly in order to ensure you foods are as flavorful as possible. Always sauté your vegetables whenever possible in order to get the fullest flavors. In addition, consider trying spicier foods than you are typically used to as the flavors will blend and mellow more than with other types of preparation.

Chapter 2: Slow Cooker Vegan Chili

Bulgur Chili

This recipe makes 6 servings and requires about 15 minutes of preparation and 8 hours of cooking on a low heat.

What's in It

- Black pepper (to taste)

- Salt (to taste)

- Cayenne pepper (to taste)

- Oregano (1 tsp. dried)

- Cumin (2 tsp.)

- Chili powder (2 T)

- Cocoa powder (1 T)

- Brown sugar (2 T)

- Pinto beans (14 oz. drained)

- Kidney beans (14 oz. drained)

- Tomatoes (14 oz. can diced)

- Coffee (1 cup brewed)

- Vegetable broth (1 cup)

- Garlic (2 cloves minced)

- Red bell pepper (.5 cups diced)

- White button mushrooms (2 cups sliced)

- Yellow onion (2 cups diced)

- Bulgur wheat (.75 cups)

How's It Made

- Add the bulgur to a large bowl before adding boiling water (2 cups) to the bowl as well. Allow the bulgur to soak for 15 minutes before draining the bowl and squeezing the results to remove excess water.

- Combine all of the ingredients together in your slow cooker and mix well. Cover the slow cooker and let it cook on a low heat for 8 hours.

- Season as desired, serve hot and enjoy.

Pumpkin And Black Bean Chili

This recipe makes 6 servings and requires about 10 minutes of preparation and 8 hours of cooking on a low heat.

What's in It

- Black pepper (to taste)

- Salt (to taste)

- Cloves (.25 tsp. ground)

- Nutmeg (.25 tsp.)

- Cumin (1 tsp.)

- Cinnamon (1 tsp.)

- Chili powder (1 T)

- Yellow bell pepper (1 medium diced)

- Yellow onion (2 cups diced)

- Pumpkin (1 cup pureed)

- Tomatoes (29 oz. diced)

- Black beans (45 oz. drained)

How's It Made

- Combine all of the ingredients together in a slow cooker that is at least 4-quarts and mix well.

- Cover the slow cooker and let it cook on a low heat for 8 hours.

- Season as desired, serve hot and enjoy.

Cauliflower Chili

This recipe makes 6 servings and requires about 15 minutes of preparation and 8 hours of cooking on a low heat.

What's in It

- Black pepper (to taste)

- Salt (to taste)

- Cayenne pepper (to taste)

- Cumin (2 tsp.)

- Chili powder (1 T)

- Brown sugar (2 T)

- Hot sauce (.5 cups)

- Green chilies (4 oz. diced)

- Tomatoes (28 oz. can diced, in juice)

- Cannellini beans (4 cups cooked)

- White onion (2 cups diced)

- Cauliflower (4 cups florets)

How's It Made

- Combine all of the ingredients together in a slow cooker that is at least 3-quarts and mix well.

- Cover the slow cooker and let it cook on a low heat for at least 8 hours.

- Season as desired, serve hot and enjoy.

Mango And Black Bean Chili

This recipe makes 6 servings and requires about 15 minutes of preparation and 8 hours of cooking on a low heat.

What's in It

- Black pepper (to taste)

- Salt (to taste)

- Mango (2 cups diced)

- Allspice (.25 tsp.)

- Cinnamon (.5 tsp.)

- Paprika (.5 tsp.)

- Cumin (1 tsp.)

- Chili powder (1 T)

- Golden raisins (. 5 cups)

- Orange juice (.5 cups)

- Black beans (4 cups cooked)

- Tomatoes (28 oz. diced)

- Jalapeno pepper (1 diced)

- Garlic (3 cloves minced)

- Yellow onion (2 cups diced)

How's It Made

- Combine all of the ingredients, besides the mangoes) together in a slow cooker that is at least 3-quarts and mix well.

- Cover the slow cooker and let it cook on a low heat for at least 8 hours.

- Add in the mango and mix well before letting the slow cooker cook for another 10 minutes.

- Season as desired, serve hot and enjoy.

Black Bean, Sweet Potato And Quinoa Chili

This recipe makes 6 servings and requires about 15 minutes of preparation and 8 hours of cooking on a low heat.

What's in It

- Black pepper (to taste)
- Salt (to taste)
- Cayenne pepper (to taste)
- Paprika (.25 tsp. smoked)
- Cumin (2 tsp.)
- Chili powder (1 T)
- Cocoa powder (2 T)
- Sweet potatoes (2 diced, peeled)
- Jalapeno pepper (1 minced, seeded)
- Green bell pepper (1 diced)
- Tomatoes (28 oz. diced)
- Vegetable broth (2 cups)
- Black beans (3 cups cooked)
- Quinoa (.5 cups)

How's It Made

- Combine all of the ingredients together in a slow cooker that is at least 3-quarts and mix well.

- Cover the slow cooker and let it cook on a low heat for at least 8 hours.

- Season as desired, serve hot and enjoy.

Red Lentil And Pumpkin Chili

This recipe makes 6 servings and requires about 10 minutes of preparation and 8 hours of cooking on a low heat.

What's in It

- Black pepper (to taste)

- Salt (to taste)

- Cloves (.25 tsp.)

- Cinnamon (.5 tsp.)

- Cumin (2 tsp.)

- Chili powder (1 T)

- Cocoa powder (1 T)

- Jalapeno pepper (1 minced, seeded)

- Yellow onion (1 cup chopped)

- Pumpkin puree (1 cup)

- Red lentils (1 cup)

- Diced tomatoes (30 oz.)

- Vegetable broth (2 cups)

- Kidney beans (30 oz. drained)

How's It Made

- Combine all of the ingredients together in a slow cooker that is at least 3-quarts and mix well.

- Cover the slow cooker and let it cook on a low heat for at least 8 hours.

- Season as desired, serve hot and enjoy.

3 Bean Chili

This recipe makes 6 servings and requires about 15 minutes of preparation and 8 hours of cooking on a low heat.

What's in It

- Black pepper (to taste)

- Salt (to taste)

- Tabasco sauce (to taste)

- Oregano (1 tsp.)

- Cumin (1 T)

- Chili powder (2 T)

- Garlic (2 cloves chopped)

- Yellow onion (3 cups chopped)

- Green peppers (3 cups chopped)

- Tomatoes (28 oz. diced)

- Black beans (15 oz. drained)

- Kidney beans (15 oz. drained)

- Chili beans (30 oz. in sauce)

How's It Made

- Combine all of the ingredients together in a slow cooker that is at least 4-quarts and mix well.

- Cover the slow cooker and let it cook on a low heat for at least 8 hours.

- Season as desired, serve hot and enjoy.

Poblanos And Quinoa White Chili

This recipe makes 8 servings and requires about 15 minutes of preparation and 8 hours of cooking on a low heat.

What's in It

- Black pepper (to taste)

- Salt (to taste)

- Tabasco (to taste)

- Quinoa (.75 cups, rinsed, drained)

- Cannellini beans (4 cups cooked)

- Vegetable broth (3 cups)

- Cloves (.25 tsp. ground)

- Paprika (.25 tsp. smoked)

- Oregano (1 tsp. dried)

- Cumin (2 tsp.)

- Garlic (2 cloves minced)

- Green pepper (1.5 cups diced)

- White onion (2 cups diced)

- Olive oil (1 T)

- Poblano peppers (.5 lbs.)

How's It Made

- Ensure you oven is set to high broil before placing the rack less than halfway from the oven's top.

- Add the pepper to a cookie sheet before adding them to the oven and letting them cook for 2 minutes until one side starts to blacken before repeating with the remaining sides.

- After removing the peppers from the oven, cover them with foil before letting them cool.

- Add the olive oil to a pan before placing it on the stove above a burner turned to a high/medium heat. Add the green peppers and diced onions to the pan and let them cook for 5 minutes.

- Mix the salt, cloves, paprika, cumin, oregano and garlic into the pan and stir for 60 seconds before adding in 1 cup of broth and mixing well. Add the results as well as the Tabasco sauce, quinoa, cannellini beans and remaining vegetable broth to the slow cooker.

- Peel the peppers and dice them, removing the seeds as desired before adding them to the slow cooker and mixing well.

- Cover the slow cooker and let it cook on a low heat for 8 hours.

- Season as desired, serve hot and enjoy.

Classic Chili

This recipe makes 4 servings and requires about 10 minutes of preparation and 8 hours of cooking on a low heat.

What's in It

- Black pepper (to taste)

- Salt (to taste)

- Hot sauce (to taste)

- Cayenne pepper 9.5 tsp.)

- Oregano (1 tsp.)

- Paprika (1 T smoked)

- Cumin (1 T)

- Chili powder (2 T)

- Brown sugar (3 T)

- Garlic (4 cloves minced)

- Jalapeno pepper (.5 minced, seeded)

- Red bell pepper (1 diced)

- Onion (1 diced)

- Coffee (.5 cups brewed)

- Kidney beans (15 oz. drained)

- Black beans (15 oz. drained)

- Tomatoes (28 oz. diced, drained)

How's It Made

- Combine all of the ingredients together in a slow cooker that is at least 3-quarts and mix well.

- Cover the slow cooker and let it cook on a low heat for at least 8 hours.

- Season as desired, serve hot and enjoy.

Butter Nut Squash Chili

This recipe makes 4 servings and requires about 10 minutes of preparation and 8 hours of cooking on a low heat.

What's in It

- Black pepper (to taste)

- Salt (to taste)

- Oregano (1 tsp.)

- Paprika (1 T smoked)
- Chili powder (1 T)
- Cumin (2 T)
- Chipotle peppers in Adobo (2 minced, seeded)
- Garlic (3 cloves minced)
- Corn (1 cup kernels)
- Vegetable broth 92 cups)
- Butternut squash (4 cups diced, peeled)
- Kidney beans (14 oz. drained)
- Tomatoes (14 oz. diced)
- Red pepper (diced, seeded)
- White onion (1 diced)

How's It Made

- Combine all of the ingredients together in a slow cooker that is at least 4-quarts and mix well.
- Cover the slow cooker and let it cook on a low heat for at least 8 hours.
- Season as desired, serve hot and enjoy.

Tempeh Chili

This recipe makes 12 servings and requires about 20 minutes of preparation and 6 hours of cooking on a low heat.

What's in It

- Black pepper (to taste)
- Salt (to taste)
- Flat leaf parsley (.5 cups chopped)
- Nutmeg (.5 tsp. divided)
- Paprika (.5 tsp smoked, divided)
- Cumin (1 tsp. ground, divided)
- Chili powder (1 tsp. divided)
- Cayenne pepper (1 tsp. divided)
- Black beans (15 oz.)
- Kidney beans (15 oz.)
- Vegetable broth (1 cup)
- Tomatoes (28 oz. diced)
- Tempeh (8 oz. cubed)
- Yellow onion (1 cup diced)
- Beet (1 cup cubed, peeled)
- Carrots (1 cup cubed, peeled)
- Parsnips (2 cups cubed, peeled)
- Sweet potatoes (2 cups cubed, peeled)
- Turnips (2 cups cubed, peeled)

- Rutabagas (2 cups cubed, peeled)

How's It Made

- In the slow cooker, add the vegetables and mix well to create a bottom layer. Add a layer of tempeh before adding in the diced tomatoes, beans and vegetable broth.

- Cover the slow cooker and let it cook on a low heat for 2 hours before adding in 50 percent of the seasonings. After 4 additional hours, mix in the reaming seasonings.

- Season as desired, serve hot and enjoy.

Chapter 3: Slow Cooker Vegan Soups

Brown Rice And Black Bean Soup

This recipe makes 6 servings and requires about 20 minutes of preparation and 7 hours of cooking on a low heat.

What's in It

- Black pepper (to taste)

- Salt (to taste)

- Brown rice (2 cups cooked)

- Tabasco sauce (to taste)

- Tomato paste (2 T)

- Vegetable broth (4 cups)

- Oregano (1 tsp. dried)

- Cumin (1 tsp.)

- Chili powder (1 tsp.)

- Garlic (1 T minced)

- Jalapeno pepper (1 diced, seeds removed)

- Carrot (1 cup diced)

- Yellow onion (1 cup diced)

- Olive oil (1 T)

- Black beans (45 oz. drained + 15 oz.)

How's It Made

- Add 45 oz. of beans to a slow cooker, that is at least 3-quarts.

- Add the olive oil to a pan before adding the pan to the stove over a burner turned to a medium heat. Add in the carrots and onion before letting them cook for 5 minutes. Mix in the pepper, salt, oregano, cumin, chili powder, garlic, pepper and jalapeno before stirring well for 60 seconds. Mix in the tabasco sauce, vegetable broth and tomato paste and stir well before adding the results to the slow cooker.

- Cover the slow cooker and let it cook on a low heat for at least 6 hours.

- Blend results before adding the remaining beans and the soup to the slow cooker and letting it cook on low for an additional hour.

- Season as desired, serve hot and enjoy.

Minestrone

This recipe makes 8 servings and requires about 35 minutes of preparation and 6 hours of cooking on a low heat.

What's in It

- Black pepper (to taste)

- Salt (to taste)

- Spinach (4 cups chopped)

- Elbow macaroni (.5 cups)

- Thyme (.75 tsp. dried)

- Oregano (1.5 tsp. dried)

- Parsley (1 T minced)

- Garlic (3 cloves minced)

- Zucchini (1 small chopped, peeled)

- Green beans (1 cup)

- Carrots (2 diced, peeled)

- Celery (2 ribs, diced, peeled)

- Yellow onion (1 chopped)

- Kidney beans (15 oz. drained)

- Tomatoes (28 oz. crushed)

- Vegetable broth (6 cups)

How's It Made

- Add the salt, black pepper, thyme, oregano, parsley, garlic, zucchini, green beans, carrots, celery, onion, kidney beans, tomatoes and vegetable broth to a slow cooker that is at least 4-quarts. Cover the slow cooker and let it cook on a low heat for at least 6 hours.

- Blend results using an immersion blender.

- Add the elbow macaroni into the slow cooker and let everything cook for an additional 20 minutes. Add in the spinach 5 minutes prior to serving.

- Season as desired, serve hot and enjoy.

Corn Chowder

This recipe makes 6 servings and requires about 30 minutes of preparation and 8 hours and 2o minutes of cooking on a low heat.

What's in It

- Black pepper (to taste)

- Salt (to taste)

- Almond milk (1 cup)

- Kosher salt (1 tsp.)

- Cayenne pepper (.25 tsp.)

- Paprika (.5 tsp. smoked)

- Cumin (1 tsp.)

- Vegetable broth (4 cups)

- Corn (4 cups kernels)

- Red bell pepper (diced, seeded)

- Yellow onion (2 cups diced)

- Olive oil (2 T)

How's It Made

- Add the olive oil to a pan before adding the pan to the stove over a burner turned to a medium heat. Place the onions in the pan and let them cook until the onion becomes transparent.

- Add the salt, cayenne pepper, smoked paprika, cumin, vegetable broth, one fourth of the corn, the potatoes and red bell pepper to the slow cooker and mix well.

- Cover the slow cooker and let it cook on a low heat for at least 8 hours.

- Use an immersion blender to blend the cooked soup before adding in the remaining corn and soy milk, recovering the slow cooker and letting it cook for an additional 20 minutes

- Season as desired, serve hot and enjoy.

Classic Vegetable Soup

This recipe makes 6 servings and requires about 15 minutes of preparation and 6 hours of cooking on a low heat.

What's in It

- Black pepper (to taste)

- Salt (to taste)

- Garlic powder (2 T)

- Rosemary (2.5 T dried)

- Olive oil (6 T)

- Black beans (15 oz. drained)

- Kidney beans (15 oz. drained)

- Vegetable broth (8 cups)

- Tomatoes (28 oz. diced)

- Onions (12 oz. chopped)

- Carrots (16 oz. chopped)

- Cauliflower (16 oz. florets)

- Broccoli (16 oz. chopped)

How's It Made

- Combine all of the ingredients together in a slow cooker that is at least 5-quarts and mix well.

- Cover the slow cooker and let it cook on a low heat for at least 6 hours before using an emersion blender to blend well.

- Season as desired, serve hot and enjoy.

Chinese Soup

This recipe makes 8 servings and requires about 30 minutes of preparation and 8 hours of cooking on a low heat.

What's in It-Soup

- Black pepper (to taste)
- Salt (to taste)
- Vegetable stock (60 oz.)
- Soy sauce (3 T)
- Red pepper flakes (.5 tsp.)
- Ginger paste (2 T)
- Garlic paste (2 T)
- Bamboo shoots (8 oz.)
- Water chestnuts (8 oz. sliced)
- Celery stalks (2 chopped)
- Carrot (1 cup chopped)
- Yellow onion (1 chopped)
- Scallions (6 chopped)
- Snow peas (1 oz. sliced)
- White button mushrooms (4 oz. sliced)
- Tofu (8 oz. cubed, drained)
- Bok choy (2 bunches sliced)

What's in It-Sauce

- Soy sauce (2 T)
- Sesame oil (1 tsp.)

- Agave syrup (2 T)
- Ginger paste (2 T)

How's It Made

- Combine the vegetable stock, soy sauce, red pepper flakes, ginger paste, garlic paste, bamboo shoots, water chestnuts, celery stalks, carrots, and yellow onion in a slow cooker that is at least 5-quarts and mix well.

- Cover the slow cooker and let it cook on a low heat for at least 7 hours before adding the remaining ingredients and cooking for another hour before using an emersion blender to blend well.

- Combine the sauce ingredients tighter to make the sauce, season as desired, serve hot and enjoy.

Lentil, Potato And Chard Soup

This recipe makes 6 servings and requires about 20 minutes of preparation and 8 hours of cooking on a low heat.

What's in It

- Salt (to taste)
- Black pepper (to taste)
- Soy sauce (1 T)
- Vegetable broth (6 cups)
- Potatoes (4 chopped)

- Brown lentils (1 cup dried)

- Swiss Chard (1 bunch torn)

- Garlic cloves (2 minced)

- Carrot (1 sliced)

- Celery stalk (1 sliced)

- Yellow onion (1 chopped)

- Olive oil (1 T)

How's It Made

- Add the oil to a skillet before adding the skillet to the stove over a burner turned to a medium heat. Add in the chard stems, garlic, carrot, celery and onion before covering the skillet and letting it cook for 8 minutes stirring once per minute.

- Add the results as well as the soy sauce, vegetable broth, potatoes and lentils to a slow cooker that is at least 6-quarts and mix well.

- Cover the slow cooker and let it cook on a low heat for at least 8 hours.

- Prior to the majority of the soup finishing, add water and a pinch of salt to a large pot of water before adding it to the stove over a burner turned to a high heat. After the water boils add in the chard and let it cook for 5 minutes.

- Add the chad to the slow cooker and use an immersion blender to blend soup to the desired consistency.

- Season as desired, serve hot and enjoy.

Chickpea And Red Lentil Soup

This recipe makes 8 servings and requires about 15 minutes of preparation and 4 hours of cooking on a high heat.

What's in It

- Salt (to taste)

- Black pepper (to taste)

- Tomatoes (28 oz. diced)

- Vegetable stock (5 cups)

- Chickpeas (30 oz. rinsed)

- Red lentils (1 cup)

- Thyme (.5 tsp. dried)

- Paprika (2 tsp. smoked)

- Garlic (1 T minced)

- Olive oil (1 T)

- Yellow onion (1 diced)

How's It Made

- Add the olive oil to a skillet before placing it on the stove over a burner turned to a high/medium heat. Add in the onion and let it cook for 5 minutes before adding in the pepper, salt, thyme, paprika and garlic and letting everything cook for 2 additional minutes.

- Add the results to a slow cooker that is at least 3.5-quarts. Before adding in the vegetable stock, chickpeas and red lentils, covering the slow cooker and letting it cook for 2 hours on a high heat.

- After 2 hours, add in the diced tomatoes before cooking for an additional 2 hours before using an emersion blender to blend well.

- Season as desired, serve hot and enjoy.

Mixed Bean Soup

This recipe makes 6 servings and requires about 10 minutes of preparation and 6 hours of cooking on a low heat.

What's in It

- Salt (to taste)

- Black pepper (to taste)

- Thyme (1 T)

- Vegetable stock (7 cups)

- Garlic (4 cloves minced)

- Carrots (4 chopped)

- Onion (1 chopped)

- Grain and bean soup mix (1.5 cups)

How's It Made

- Use a bowl of water to soak the soup mix overnight prior to making the soup.

- Combine all of the ingredients together in a slow cooker that is at least 5-quarts and mix well.

- Cover the slow cooker and let it cook on a low heat for at least 8 hours before using an emersion blender to blend well.

- Season as desired, serve hot and enjoy.

Thai Curry Soup

This recipe makes 6 servings and requires about 15 minutes of preparation and 8 hours of cooking on a low heat.

What's in It

- Salt (to taste)

- Black pepper (to taste)

- Thai red curry paste (3 T)

- Coconut milk (14 oz.)

- Vegetable broth (4 cups)

- Yellow onion (1 diced)

- Butternut squash (8 cups cubed)

How's It Made

- Combine all of the ingredients together except for the Thai red curry paste and coconut milk in a slow cooker that is at least 4-quarts and mix well.

- Cover the slow cooker and let it cook on a low heat for at least 7.5 hours before using an emersion blender to blend well then mixing in the Thai red curry paste as well as the coconut milk. Recover the slow cooker and let it cook for an additional 30 minutes.

- Season as desired, serve hot and enjoy.

Summer Squash And White Bean Soup

This recipe makes 4 servings and requires about 20 minutes of preparation and 8 hours and 30 minutes of cooking on a low heat.

What's in It

- Salt (to taste)

- Black pepper (to taste)

- Basil (7 leaves torn)

- Water (4 cups)

- Paprika (.5 tsp. smoked)

- Italian seasoning (2 tsp.)

- Garlic (2 cloves minced)

- Yellow onion (1 cup diced)

- Potato (1.5 cups diced)

- Summer squash (2 cups diced)

- Tomatoes (14.5 oz. diced)

- Cannelloni beans (14.5 oz. drained)

How's It Made

- Combine all of the ingredients except the basil leaves together in a slow cooker that is at least 3.5-quarts and mix well.

- Cover the slow cooker and let it cook on a low heat for at least 8 hours before using an emersion blender to blend well.

- Add in the basil leaves, season as desired, serve hot and enjoy.

Veggie Pasta Soup

This recipe makes 6 servings and requires about 15 minutes of preparation and 8 hours of cooking on a low heat.

What's in It

- Salt (to taste)

- Black pepper (to taste)

- Red wine vinegar (2 T)

- Pasta (1 cup)

- Tomatoes (14 oz.)

- Kidney beans (15 oz. drained)

- Zucchini (1 diced)

- Carrots (1 cup peeled, diced)

- Cabbage (4 cups chopped)

- Vegetable broth (4 cups)

- Italian seasoning (2 tsp.)

- Garlic (2 cloves minced)

- Onion (1 diced)

- Olive oil (2 tsp.)

How's It Made

- Add the olive oil to a skillet before adding the skillet to the stove turned to a medium heat. Mix in the onions and let them cook for 6 minutes before adding in the pepper, salt, Italian seasoning and letting everything cook for 1 minute. Add in .5 cups of broth before adding the results to the slow cooker that is at least 4-quarts.

- Mix in the remaining broth as well as the tomatoes, beans, zucchini, carrots and cabbage. Cover the slow cooker and let it cook on a low heat for at least

7.5 hours before using an emersion blender to blend well. Add in the pasta, recover and let it cook for 30 minutes.

- Add in the red wine vinegar, season as desired, serve hot and enjoy.

Cauliflower Soup With Split Pea

This recipe makes 8 servings and requires about 10 minutes of preparation and 6 hours of cooking on a low heat.

What's in It

- Salt (to taste)

- Black pepper (to taste)

- Bay leaf (1 torn)

- Thyme (.5 tsp.)

- Sage (.5 tsp.)

- Cumin (1 tsp.)

- Vegetable broth (6 cups)

- Split peas (2 cups dried)

- Cauliflower (3 cups chopped)

- Garlic (2 cloves minced)

- Celery (1 stalk diced)

- Onion (2 cups diced)

- Olive oil (1 T)

How's It Made

- Add the olive oil to a pan before adding the pan to the stove over a burner turned to a medium heat and adding in the celery and onion before letting them cook for 5 minutes. Add in the garlic and let it cook for 60 seconds.

- Combine all of the ingredients together in a slow cooker that is at least 4.5-quarts and mix well.

- Cover the slow cooker and let it cook on a low heat for at least 8 hours before using an emersion blender to blend well.

- Season as desired, serve hot and enjoy.

Chapter 4: Slow Cooker Vegan Curries

Red Lentil, Chickpea And Pumpkin Curry

This recipe makes 6 servings and requires about 10 minutes of preparation and 8 hours of cooking on a low heat.

What's in It

- Salt (to taste)

- Black pepper (to taste)

- Coconut milk (15 oz.)

- Cayenne pepper (.25 tsp.)

- Curry powder (1 T)

- Pumpkin puree (1 cup)

- Red lentils (1 cup rinsed)

- Vegetable broth (2 cups)

- Garlic (2 cloves minced)

- Yellow onion (1 diced)

- Chickpeas (30 oz. drained)

How's It Made

- Combine all of the ingredients together save the coconut milk in a slow cooker that is at least 3-quarts and mix well.

- Cover the slow cooker and let it cook on a low heat for at least 8 hours. 30 minutes prior to completion, add in the coconut milk.

- Serve over cauliflower rice as desired, season, serve hot and enjoy.

Chickpea Curry

This recipe makes 6 servings and requires about 10 minutes of preparation and 8 hours of cooking on a low heat.

What's in It

- Salt (to taste)

- Chickpeas (30 oz. drained)

- Tomatoes (whole, peeled, in juice 28 oz.)

- Cayenne powder (.25 tsp.)

- Coriander (.5 tsp. ground)

- Garam masala (1 tsp.)

- Cumin (2 tsp.)

- Cardamom 3 pods, seeded, crushed)

- Ginger (1 T mined)

- Garlic (3 cloves minced)

- Yellow onion (1 diced)

- Olive oil (2 T)

How's It Made

- Add the olive oil to a skillet before placing it on the stove over a burner turned to a medium heat.

- Mix in the onions and let them cook for 7 minutes before adding in the garlic and letting it cook for an additional minute.

- Mix in the salt, cayenne powder, coriander, Garam masala, cumin, cardamom and ginger before letting them cook for 30 seconds. Add in the tomatoes and mix well.

- Add the results to a slow cooker that is at least 4-quarts before adding in the chickpeas and mixing well.

- Cover the slow cooker and let it cook on a low heat for at least 8 hours.

- Serve over cauliflower rice as desired, season, serve hot and enjoy.

Curried Potatoes With Chickpeas

This recipe makes 4 servings and requires about 20 minutes of preparation and 4 hours of cooking on a low heat.

What's in It

- Salt (to taste)

- Chickpeas (30 oz. drained)

- Cilantro (1 bunch chopped)
- Lime (1)
- Red potatoes (1 lb. diced)
- Vegetable broth (1 cup)
- Tomato paste (2 T)
- Tomatoes (14 oz. diced)
- Red pepper flakes (.25 tsp.)
- Turmeric (.25 tsp.)
- Ginger (.5 tsp. ground)
- Garam masala (.5 tsp.)
- Cumin (2 tsp.)
- Coriander (2 tsp.)
- Garlic (2 cloves minced)
- Yellow onion (2 cups diced)
- Olive oil (2 tsp.)

How's It Made

- Add the olive oil to the pan before adding the pan to the stove over a burner turned to a medium heat. Add in the onion and let it cook for 5 minutes before adding in the salt, red pepper flakes, turmeric, ground ginger, Garam masala, cumin, coriander and garlic. Stir well and let the results cook for a minute.

- Mix in the vegetable broth and tomato paste and stir well before adding the results to a slow cooker that is at least 3-quarts and mix well before adding the remaining ingredients

- Cover the slow cooker and let it cook on a low heat for at least 8 hours.

- Serve over cauliflower rice as desired, season, serve hot and enjoy.

Lentil Dal

This recipe makes 12 servings and requires about 10 minutes of preparation and 5 hours of cooking on a low heat.

What's in It

- Salt (to taste)

- Lemon juice (to taste)

- Cilantro (to taste)

- Black pepper (.25 tsp.)

- Fennel seeds (1 tsp.)

- Cumin seeds (2 tsp.)

- Mustard seeds (2 tsp.)

- Onion seeds (2 tsp.)

- Fenugreek seeds (2 tsp.)

- Bay leaf (1 torn)

- Cardamom pods (3)

- Turmeric (1 T)

- Ginger (2 T)

- Garlic (4 cloves minced)

- Onion (1 diced)

- Tomatoes (28 oz. diced)

- Red lentils (1.5 cups)

- Spilt peas (1.5 cups

How's It Made

- Add the split peas and the lentils to a mixing bowl before filling the bowl with water and letting them soak for 10 minutes. Rise the beans after draining them before adding them to the slow cooker that is at least 4-quarts before adding in the black pepper, salt, bay leaf, cardamom pods, turmeric, ginger, garlic, onion, tomatoes and 6 cups of water.

- Add the cumin seeds, fenugreek seeds, onion seeds and mustard seeds to a skillet before placing that skillet on the stove over a medium heat. Toast the seeds until they begin to be fragrant before adding them to the slow cooker.

- Cover the slow cooker and let it cook on a low heat for at least 8 hours.

- Serve over cauliflower rice as desired, season, serve hot and enjoy.

Lentil Curry

This recipe makes 8 servings and requires about 10 minutes of preparation and 6 hours of cooking on a low heat.

What's in It

- Salt (to taste)

- Cilantro (.25 cups chopped)

- Lime juice (1 T)

- Sugar (2 tsp.)

- Cayenne pepper (.5 tsp.)

- Cumin (.5 tsp.)

- Coriander (.5 tsp. ground)

- Curry paste (2 T)

- Vegetable broth (4 cups)

- Ginger (1 tsp. ground)

- Garlic (1 T minced)

- Yellow onion (1 chopped)

- Tomatoes (14 oz. diced)

- Cauliflower (2 cups florets)

- Spinach (10 oz.)

- Red lentils (2 cups)

How's It Made

- Add all of the ingredients save the cilantro and lime juice to a slow cooker that is at least 3-quarts.

- Cover the slow cooker and let it cook on a low heat for at least 8 hours.

- Serve over cauliflower rice as desired, season with lime juice and cilantro, serve hot and enjoy.

Tofu Curry

This recipe makes 6 servings and requires about 10 minutes of preparation and 6 hours of cooking on a low heat.

What's in It

- Salt (to taste)

- Black pepper (to taste)

- Cilantro (3 T chopped)

- Canola oil 91 T)

- Tofu (14 oz. drained)

- Coconut milk (13.5 oz.)

- Tomatoes (14 oz. in juice, diced)

- Chickpeas (16 oz. drained)

- Garlic (2 cloves minced)

- Salt (1.25 tsp.)

- Ginger (1 T grated)

- Brown sugar (1 T)

- Curry powder (1 T)

- Yellow onion (1 cup chopped)

- Cauliflower (2 cups florets)

- Sweet potato (2 cups cubed)

How's It Made

- Add the sweet potato cubes, the cauliflower florets, the chopped onion, the curry powder, brown sugar, ginger, salt, garlic, chickpeas, tomatoes, coconut milk and to a slow cooker that is at least 4-quarts. Cover the slow cooker and let it cook for 5.5 hours.

- Add the olive oil to a skillet before placing it on the stove over a burner turned to a high/medium heat. Add in the tofu and let it cook for 8 minutes before adding it to the slow cooker and letting it cook for 30 minutes.

- Serve over cauliflower rice as desired, season, serve hot and enjoy.

Classic Curry With Vegetables

This recipe makes 8 servings and requires about 15 minutes of preparation and 6 hours of cooking on a low heat.

What's in It

- Salt (to taste)

- Coconut milk (.5 cups)

- Peas 9.5 cups)

- Vegetable stock (2 cups)

- Tomatoes (1 cup diced)

- Chickpeas (3 cups drained)

- Red potatoes (4 quartered)

- Turmeric (.5 tsp.)

- Garam masala (.5 tsp.)

- Cumin (1 tsp.)

- Curry powder (2 T)

- Garlic (3 cloves sliced)

- Onion (1 sliced)

- Carrots (2 cups sliced)

- Canola oil (1 T)

How's It Made

- Add the canola oil to a skillet before adding the skillet to the stove over a burner turned to a medium heat. Add in the onion as well as the carrots and let them cook for 3 minutes before mixing in the turmeric, Garam masala, cumin, curry powder and garlic and letting everything cook for 2 minutes.

- Add the results to a slow cooker that is at least 3-quarts before adding in the vegetable stock, tomatoes, chickpeas, green beans and potatoes as well.

- Cover the slow cooker and let it cook on a low heat for at least 5.5 hours before adding in the coconut milk and the peas and letting them cook for 30 minutes.

- Serve over cauliflower rice as desired, season, serve hot and enjoy.

Sweet Potato Curry

This recipe makes 8 servings and requires about 15 minutes of preparation and 6 hours of cooking on a low heat.

What's in It

- Salt (to taste)

- Spinach leaves (1.5 cups chopped)

- Coconut milk (.5 cups)

- Ground pepper (.5 tsp.)

- Vegetable broth (14 oz.)

- Tomatoes (14 oz. diced)

- Chickpeas (2.5 cups)

- Cauliflower (2 cups florets)

- Sweet potato (2 cups diced)

- Curry paste (.25 cups)

- Garlic (2 cloves minced)

- Gala apple (1 diced)

- Yellow onion (.5 diced)

- Canola oil (1 tsp.)

How's It Made

- Add the oil to a pan before adding the pan to the stove over a burner turned to a medium heat. Add in the ginger, apple and onion and let them cook for 7 minutes.

- Mix in the garlic and let it cook briefly before adding the curry paste and letting it cook for 3 minutes, stirring constantly.

- Add the results to a slow cooker that is at least 3-quarts before adding in the vegetable broth, diced tomatoes, chickpeas, cauliflower and sweet potato.

- Cover the slow cooker and let it cook on a low heat for at least 6 hours.

- Add in the spinach and coconut milk, mix well, serve over cauliflower rice as desired, season, serve hot and enjoy.

Yellow Curry

This recipe makes 8 servings and requires about 15 minutes of preparation and 8 hours of cooking on a low heat.

What's in It

- Salt (to taste)

- Lemongrass (1 tsp. inner core chopped)

- Garlic (3 cloves minced)

- Ginger (1 T minced)

- Coriander (1 tsp.)

- Turmeric (1 tsp.)

- Cumin (.5 tsp.)

- Garam masala (1 tsp.)

- Coconut milk (15 oz.)

- Vegetable broth (.75 cups)

- Golden raisins (1 cup)

- Peas (1 cup)

- Carrots (2 cups chopped, peeled)

- Potatoes (2 cups diced)

- Sweet onion (2 cups chopped)

- Orange bell pepper (.5 cups chopped)

- Chickpeas (15 oz. drained)

How's It Made

- Add all of the ingredients to a slow cooker that is at least 3-quarts

- Cover the slow cooker and let it cook on a low heat for at least 8 hours.

- Serve over cauliflower rice as desired, season, serve hot and enjoy.

Green Curry

This recipe makes 4 servings and requires about 30 minutes of preparation and 8 hours of cooking on a low heat.

What's in It

- Salt (to taste)

- Eggplant (1 chopped)

- Peas (.75 cups)

- Bell pepper (1.5 cups sliced)

- Yellow onion (1 chopped)

- Coconut sugar (1 T)

- Turmeric (.5 tsp.)

- Ginger (1 T minced)

- Green curry paste (.25 cups)

- Vegetable broth (1 cup)

- Coconut milk (14.5 oz.)

- Tofu (16 oz. pressed, drained, diced)

How's It Made

- Add the coconut sugar, salt, turmeric, ginger, curry paste, vegetable broth, and coconut milk to a slow cooker that is at least 4-quarts and mix well.

- Add in everything save the tofu and cover the slow cooker and let it cook on a low heat for at least 6 hours.

- Add the oil to a pan before adding the pan to the stove over a burner turned to a medium heat. Add in the tofu and let it cook for 4 minutes per side.

- Add the tofu to the curry when it has 30 minutes left to cook.

- Serve over cauliflower rice as desired, season, serve hot and enjoy.

Chapter 5: Regional Slow Cooker Vegan Favorites

Black-Eyed Peas

This recipe makes 2 servings and requires about 15 minutes of preparation and 9 hours of cooking on a low heat.

What's in It

- Salt (to taste)

- Liquid smoke (to taste)

- Cajun seasoning (1 tsp.)

- Garlic (1 clove minced)

- Bell pepper (2 T minced)

- Millet (.25 cups)

- Carrots (.3 cups chopped)

- Black-eyed peas (.3 cups dry)

- Water (2 cups)

- Tomato paste (2 T)

- Collard greens (1 cup)

How's It Made

- In a slow cooker that is at least 5-quarts, add in the liquid smoke, Cajun seasoning, garlic, bell pepper, millet, carrots, black-eyed peas and water and mix well.

- Cover your slow cooker and let it cook for 9 hours.

- Half an hour prior to serving, add in the tomato paste as well as the collard greens and mix well.

- Season as needed, serve hot and enjoy.

Slow Cooker Quinoa

This recipe makes 4 servings and requires about 5 minutes of preparation and 3 hours of cooking on a high heat.

What's in It

- Salt (to taste)

- Vegetable broth (2 cups)

- Chipotle pepper adobo sauce (1.5 T)

- Black pepper (to taste)

- Garlic (1 T minced)

- Cumin (.5 T)

- Onion (.5 cups chopped)

- Roma tomatoes (1 cup chopped)

- Red pepper (1 cup chopped)

- Black beans (.5 cups chopped)

- Chickpeas (.6 cups drained)

- Corn (1 cup kernels)

- Quinoa (1 cup)

How's It Made

- In a slow cooker that is at least 3 quarts, coat the inside with cooking spray before adding in the adobo sauce, pepper, salt, garlic, cumin powder, onion, tomato, red pepper, black beans, chickpeas, corn and quinoa and mixing well.

- Add in the vegetable broth and mix well before covering your slow cooker and letting it cook for 3 hours on a high heat.

- Season as needed, serve hot and enjoy.

Mexican Bowl With Brown Rice

This recipe makes 6 servings and requires about 5 minutes of preparation and 2 hours of cooking on a high heat.

What's in It-Slow Cooker

- Salt (to taste)

- Black pepper (to taste)

- Black beans (30 oz. drained)

- Green chilies (4 oz. diced, in juice)
- Green bell pepper (1 chopped)
- Red bell pepper (1 chopped)
- Onion (1 cup chopped)
- Vegetable stock (2 cups)
- Brown rice long-grain (1 cup)

What's in It-Salsa

- Black pepper (to taste)
- Salt (to taste)
- Cumin (.5 tsp.)
- Olive oil (2 T)
- Lime juice (3T)
- Avocado (1 cubed)
- Cilantro (.5 cups)
- Green onion (.5 cups sliced)
- Poblano pepper (1 diced)
- Tomato (.5 cups diced)

How's It Made

- In a slow cooker that is at least 3 quarts, add the onion, vegetable stock and rice to the slow cooker and let it cook for 90 minutes on a high heat.

- After 90 minutes has passed, ad in the black beans, green chilies, green bell pepper and red bell pepper, mixing well. Season as needed before cooking for an additional 30 minutes.

- Combine all of the salsa ingredients together and mix well before adding as needed.

- Season as needed, serve hot and enjoy.

Jackfruit Bulgogi

This recipe makes 12 servings and requires about 10 minutes of preparation and 6 hours of cooking on a low heat.

What's in It

- Salt (to taste)

- Black pepper (to taste)

- Water (.5 cups)

- Sesame oil (4 T)

- Green pear (1 chopped, cored)

- Onion (1 sliced, peeled)

- Garlic (8 cloves chopped)

- Ginger (2 T minced)

- Mirin (1 cup)

- Agave nectar (.5 cups)

- Soy sauce (.25 cups)

- Tamari (.5 cups)

- Green jackfruit (40 oz. in brine, drained)

How's It Made

- In a slow cooker that is at least 3 quarts, add in all of the ingredients.

- Cover the slow cooker and let it cook for at least 6 hours on a low heat.

- Break jackfruit apart as desired, season as needed, serve hot and enjoy.

Shepherds' Pie With Lentils

This recipe makes 6 servings and requires about 10 minutes of preparation and 6 hours of cooking on a low heat.

What's in It

- Salt (to taste)

- Black pepper (to taste)

- Sweet potatoes (4 cups)

- Peas (1 cup)

- Vegetable broth (2 cups)

- Tomatoes (400 g diced)

- Lentils (1.5 cups)

- Thyme (.5 tsp.)

- Garlic (2 cloves crushed)

- Carrots (2 diced, peeled)

- Celery (4 stalks diced)

- Olive oil (1 T)

- Yellow onion (1 diced)

How's It Made

- In a slow cooker that is at least 4 quarts, layer in the vegetable broth, tomatoes, lentils, pepper, thyme, salt, garlic, celery, carrots, olive oil and diced onion.

- Cover the slow cooker and let it cook for at least 6 hours on a low heat.

- Add to a bowl of baked sweet potatoes, season as needed, serve hot and enjoy.

Cabbage Rolls

This recipe makes 2 servings and requires about 45 minutes of preparation and 8 hours of cooking on a low heat.

What's in It

- Salt (to taste)

- Black pepper (to taste)

- Water (.25 cups)

- Marinara sauce (3 cups)

- Olive oil (1 T)

- Dill (2 T)

- Garlic (2 cloves minced)

- Golden raisins (.25 cups)

- Pine nuts (.25 cups toasted)

- Cremini mushrooms (2 oz.)

- Onion (.5 cups diced)

- Long-grain (1 cup cooked)

- Lentils (1 cup cooked)

- Cabbage (1 head, outer leaves removed)

How's It Made

- Fill a large pot with water and a pinch of salt and bring it to a rolling boil. Add in the cabbage and let it cook for 5 minutes. Drain the cabbage and remove up to 8 cabbage leaves, boil again as necessary.

- Combine the salt, olive oil, dill, garlic, raisins, pine nuts, mushrooms, onion, rice and lentils in a medium bowl.

- In a slow cooker that is at least 3 quarts, add the marinara sauce and the .25 cups of water and mix well.

- Add .5 cups of the mixture in the bowl into a cabbage leaf before rolling it like a burrito.

- Add the results to the slow cooker, cover the slow cooker and let it cook for at least 8 hours on a low heat.

- Season as needed, top with marinara sauce, serve hot and enjoy.

Bbq Vegetables With Tofu

This recipe makes 4 servings and requires about 15 minutes of preparation and 4 hours of cooking on a high heat.

What's in It-Sauce

- Salt (to taste)

- Black pepper (to taste)

- Water (2 T)

- Five spice powder (.25 tsp.)

- Molasses 92 tsp.)

- Red pepper (.25 tsp.)

- Brown mustard (1 T)

- Soy sauce (1 T)

- Rice wine vinegar (2 T)

- Hoisin sauce (.25 cups)

- Tomato sauce (8 oz.)

- Ginger root (2 tsp.)

- Garlic (3 cloves minced)

- Onion (1 minced)

What's in It-Slow Cooker

- Tofu (1 lb. drained, pressed, sliced)

- Water chestnuts (8 oz. sliced)

- Green bell pepper (.5 cubed)

- Zucchini (2 cubed)

- Broccoli (3 stalks, florets removed)

How's It Made

- Add the oil to a skillet before adding it to the stove over a burner turned to a medium/high heat. Add in the tofu and let each side cook for approximately 5 minutes until browned.

- In a slow cooker that is at least 3 quarts and has been coated with cooking spray, add in the tofu.

- Add the onion, ginger and garlic to the skillet and let it cook for 3 minutes. Add in the remaining ingredients and heat well before adding the results to the slow cooker.

- Cover the slow cooker and let it cook for at least 3 hours on a high heat.

- At the 3-hour mark, add in the remaining vegetables and stir well. Let the slow cooker cook for an additional hour.

- Season as needed, serve hot and enjoy.

Gumbo

This recipe makes 4 servings and requires about 20 minutes of preparation and 8 hours of cooking on a low heat.

What's in It

- Salt (to taste)

- Black pepper (to taste)

- Hot sauce (to taste)

- Bay leaf (1)

- Cajun seasoning (1 T)

- Okra (1 cup sliced)

- Zucchini (1 cut into semicircles)

- White button mushrooms (8 oz. quartered)

- Kidney beans (15 oz. drained)

- Tomatoes (14 oz. diced)

- Vegetable broth (2 cups)

- Flour (2 T)

- Garlic (3 cloves minced)

- Celery (2 stalks chopped)

- Green bell pepper (chopped)

- Yellow onion (1 chopped)

- Olive oil (2 T)

How's It Made

- Add half of the oil to a skillet before adding the skillet to the stove over a burner turned to a high/medium heat. Add in the garlic, celery, bell pepper and onion and let them cook for 7 minutes.

- In a slow cooker that is at least 4 quarts, add in the vegetable mixture.

- Add the remaining oil to the skillet before adding in the flour and cooking it for 4 minutes, stirring well. Add in the broth and let it boil before adding the results to the slow cooker.

- Add the remainder of the ingredients to the slow cooker, cover it and let it cook for at least 8hours on a low heat.

- Season as needed, serve hot and enjoy.

Bourbon Baked Beans

This recipe makes 8 servings and requires about 15 minutes of preparation and 16 hours of cooking on a low heat.

What's in It

- Salt (to taste)

- Black pepper (to taste)

- Apple cider vinegar (.25 cups)

- Olive oil (.25 cups)

- Molasses (.25 cups)

- Mustard (.25 cups)

- Ketchup (.25 cups)

- Water (1 cup)

- Brown sugar (1 cup)

- BBQ sauce (1 cup)

- Maple syrup (1 cup)

- Bourbon (1 cup)

- Navy beans (1 lb. presoaked)

How's It Made

- In a slow cooker that is at least 4 quarts, combine all of the ingredients and stir well.

- Cover the slow cooker and let it cook for at least 16 hours on a low heat.

- Season as needed, serve hot and enjoy.

Vegan Spaghetti

This recipe makes 4 servings and requires about 5 minutes of preparation and 2 hours of cooking on a high heat.

What's in It

- French fried onions (6 oz.)

- Spinach (10 oz.)

- Garlic (.25 tsp.)

- Parsley (2 T)

- Basil (2 T chopped)

- Tomatoes (3 cups diced)

- White button mushrooms (5 sliced)

- Red pepper (1 chopped)

- Garlic (2 cloves minced)

- Onion (.5 diced)

- Green pepper (1 chopped)

- Water (2 cups)

- Pasta (.5 package)

How's It Made

- In a slow cooker that is at least 3 quarts, combine all of the ingredients save the pasta, parsley and basil, cover the slow cooker and let it cook for 30 minutes on a low heat.

- Turn the slow cooker to a high heat and let it cook for an additional 90 minutes. When there are 20 minutes remaining, add the pasta, 15 minutes later add in the parsley.

- Season as needed, serve hot and enjoy.

Vegan Casserole

This recipe makes 8 servings and requires about 10 minutes of preparation and 4 hours of cooking on a high heat.

What's in It

- Salt (to taste)

- Black pepper (to taste)

- White button mushrooms (.5 cups sliced)

- Vegan cheese (.5 lbs.)

- Cream of mushroom soup (10.75 oz.)

- Water (2.5 cups)

- Wild rice mix (6 oz.)

- Celery (3 stalks sliced)

- Yellow onion (2 chopped)

How's It Made

- In a slow cooker that is at least 4 quarts, combine the yellow onion, celery stalks, wild rice mix, water, cream of mushroom soup, vegan cheese, white button mushrooms, pepper and salt before mixing well.

- Add a cover to the slow cooker before letting it sit and cook for between 3 and 4 hours on a high heat.

- Season as needed with additional pepper as well as salt, serve hot and enjoy.

Conclusion

Thank you again for downloading this book! I hope it was able to provide you with a wide variety of new recipes to experiment with as well as providing you further insight into the wonderful world of slow cooking. Hopefully, you have found a number of recipes that will soon be on permanent rotation in your own home. What's more, you should now feel more secure in your ability to remain vegan, even on the days when it seems like you have a million things happening at once.

The next step is to stop reading already and start planning out a shopping list to take advantage of all your new, soon to be favorites. Remember remaining vegan is a marathon, not a sprint, slow and steady wins the race.

Part 2

1. Usa Favourites

Vegan Crockpot Quinoa And Black Bean Chili

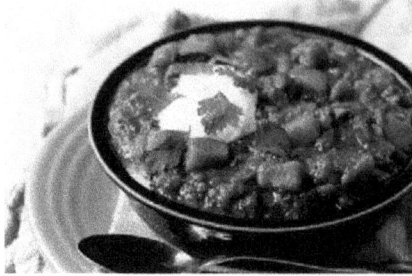

Serves: 4

Cook Time: 3 hours
Ingredients

- 2 ¼ cups vegetable broth
- ½ cup uncooked quinoa
- 15 oz can black beans, drained and rinsed
- 14 oz diced tomatoes
- ¼ cup chopped red bell pepper
- ¼ cup chopped green bell pepper
- 1 shredded carrot
- ½ onion, chopped
- 2 cloves garlic
- ½ small chili pepper

- 2 teaspoons chili powder
- ¼ teaspoon cayenne pepper
- 1 ½ teaspoon salt
- 1 teaspoon ground black pepper
- 1 teaspoon ground cumin
- 1 teaspoon oregano
- ½ cup corn kernels

Toppings

- chopped avocado chunks
- chopped green onions
- shredded carrot

Vegan Cashew Sour Cream

- ½ cup soaked cashews (cashews soaked in water overnight)
- 3-4 tablespoons water
- splash apple cider vinegar
- ½ teaspoon fine sea salt
- 1 teaspoon lime juice

Directions

1. Add the broth, quinoa, black beans and tomatoes to the slow cooker. Stir to combine.
2. Next add the peppers, carrot, onion and garlic, and stir, then add the rest of the seasonings and stir a few times to combine.

3. Set the slow cooker (Crock-Pot) to high for 2 ½ to 3 hours or on low for 5-6 hours (for high, monitor the last 30 minutes and for low, monitor the last hour). If you like a chili with more liquid, do the 2 ½ on high, and 5 on low. If you like thicker and just a little bit it liquid, go with the higher number for each option.

4. Vegan Cashew Sour Cream

5. Blend all the ingredients for cashew sour cream in a high speed blender until smooth, for about 30 seconds, scraping blender once halfway in between.

6. Serve on chili with your favourite toppings (avocado, chopped green onions).

Easy Slow Cooker Saag Aloo

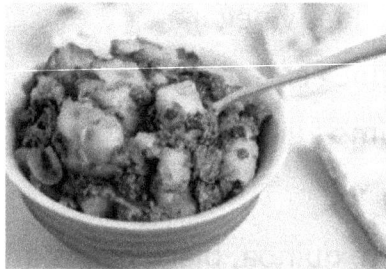

Serves: 4

Cook Time: 3 hours
Ingredients

- 650g potatoes
- ½ onion, thinly sliced
- 50ml water
- ½ vegetable stock cube, crumbled
- 1 tbsp oil
- ½ tsp cumin
- ½ tsp ground coriander
- ½ tsp garam masala
- ½ tsp hot chilli powder
- Black pepper
- 250g fresh spinach, roughly chopped

Directions

1. Peel the potatoes and cut them into chunks measuring about an inch. Add them to the slow cooker (mine›s a 3.5 litre one) along with the sliced onion, water, crumbled stock cube, oil, spices, and plenty of black pepper. Top with a couple of big handfuls of fresh spinach - however much you can easily fit in your slow cooker. I couldn›t fit all of the spinach in, so I came back and added the rest about an hour into the cooking time, once it had wilted down and created some space.

2. Cook on medium (or high if you don›t have a medium setting) for around 3 hours, until the potato is soft - stir every hour or so to scrape down the sides. The exact cooking time will depend on exactly how big you cut your potato chunks.

Slow Cooker Blueberry Butter

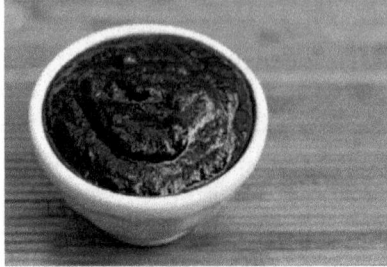

Serves: 4

Cook Time: 1 hour
Ingredients

- 36 oz. blueberries, pureed (around 5 cups of puree)
- 1 C sugar
- 2 teaspoons cinnamon
- ½ teaspoon ground nutmeg (optional)
- ¼ teaspoon ground ginger (optional)
- Zest of 1 lemon

Directions

1. Place pureed blueberries in slow cooker and turn to low. After 1 hour stir blueberry puree and prop open lid with a spatula or wooden spoon. After 4 more hours, add spices, sugar, and lemon zest. If it hasn't thickened much, remove lid and cook on high for 1 hour. Place butter in food processor or blender

and process until smooth. Store in air-tight container in fridge or in processed jars.

2. Pour into sterilized jars, leaving ½ inch of head space, wipe rims and screw on lids. Process in boiling water canner for 10 minutes. Store jars in cool, dark place.

Crockpot Sweet Potato Lentils

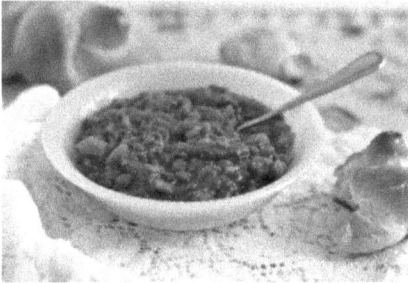

Serves: 4

Cook Time: 4.5 hours
Ingredients

- 3 large sweet potatoes, diced (about 6 cups)
- 3 cups vegetable broth
- 1 onion, minced
- 4 cloves garlic, minced
- 2 teaspoon each ground coriander, garam masala, and chili powder
- ½ teaspoon salt

- 1 ½ cups uncooked red lentils (masoor dal)
- 1 can coconut milk
- 1 cup water

Directions

1. Place the sweet potatoes, vegetable broth, onion, garlic, and spices in a crockpot. Cook on high for 3 hours, until vegetables are soft.
2. Add the lentils and stir once. Replace the lid and cook on high for an additional 1 ½ hours.
3. Stir in the coconut milk and as much water as needed to get the right consistency.

Slow Cooker Puttanesca Pizza

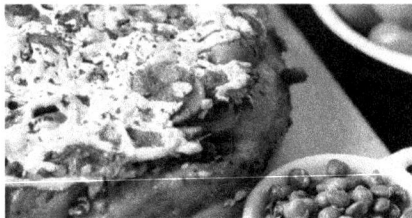

Serves: 4

Cook Time: 1.5 hours
Ingredients

For the dough:

- 1 ½ cups unbleached all-purpose flour
- 1 ½ tsp. instant yeast

- ½ tsp. salt
- ½ tsp. Italian seasoning
- 1 Tbsp. olive oil
- ½ cup warm water, or as needed

For the sauce:

- ½ cup crushed tomatoes
- ¼ cup pitted kalamata olives, sliced
- ¼ cup pitted green olives, sliced
- 1 Tbsp. capers, rinsed and drained
- 1 Tbsp. chopped fresh flat-leaf parsley
- ¼ tsp. dried basil
- ¼ tsp. dried oregano
- ¼ tsp. garlic powder
- ¼ tsp. sugar
- ¼ tsp. hot red pepper flakes
- Salt and freshly ground black pepper
- ½ cup shredded vegan mozzarella cheese (optional)

Directions

1. For the dough: Lightly oil the inside of a large bowl. In a food processor, combine the flour, yeast, salt, and Italian seasoning. With the machine running, add the oil through the feed tube, then slowly add as much water as needed to form a slightly sticky dough ball. Transfer the dough to a floured surface and knead for 1 to 2 minutes, until it is smooth and

elastic. Shape the dough into a ball and transfer to the prepared bowl, turning the dough to coat it with oil. Cover the bowl with plastic wrap and set aside to rise at warm room temperature until doubled in size, about 1 hour.

2. While the dough is rising, make the sauce. In a bowl, combine the tomatoes, both kinds of olives, capers, parsley, basil, oregano, garlic powder, sugar, red pepper flakes, and salt and black pepper to taste.

3. Generously oil the insert of a large (5- to 7-quart) slow cooker or spray it with nonstick cooking spray. Punch down the dough and transfer it to a lightly floured surface. Flatten the dough, then shape it to just fit inside your slow cooker. Place the dough in the cooker and spread the sauce over the dough. To prevent condensation from dripping onto the pizza, drape a clean kitchen towel over the cooker, then put on the lid. Cook on High for 1 hour and 45 minutes. If using the vegan mozzarella, sprinkle it on the pizza after 1 hour and 15 minutes, then cook for 30 minutes longer to allow it to melt.

White Bean Soup

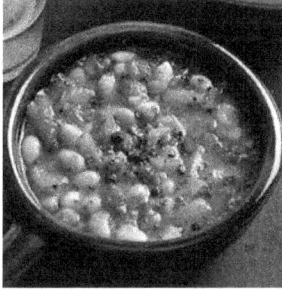

Serves: 4

Cook Time: 3 hours
Ingredients

- 1 pound dry navy beans, sorted and rinsed
- 2 quarts veggie broth
- 1 medium onion, diced
- 4 cloves of garlic, peeled and smashed
- 2 tsp salt
- ¼ tsp pepper
- 2 medium potatoes, diced
- 1 pound frozen, sliced carrots
- 1 cup chopped sun-dried tomatoes
- 1-2 tsp dried dill
- 3-4 tbsp fresh, minced parsley

Directions

1. Put the beans, veggie broth, onion, garlic, salt and pepper in a large soup pot and place over low-medium heat.
2. Allow to simmer for 3-4 hours, or longer, adding additional water as necessary.
3. When the beans are soft, but not falling apart, add the potato and continue to simmer until the potatoes are tender.
4. Add the carrots, tomatoes and dill. Keep over heat until the carrots are heated through. Stir in the parsley, season with additional salt and pepper, if needed, and serve.

Bourbon Maple Slow Cooker Baked Beans

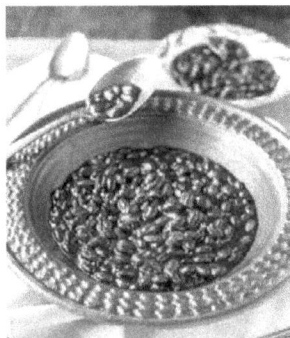

Serves: 4

Cook Time: 13 hours
Ingredients

- 1 pound dry Great Northern beans (or navy beans)
- 1 cup bourbon
- 1 cup maple syrup
- 1 cup barbeque sauce
- 1 cup light brown sugar, packed
- 1 cup water
- heaping ¼ cup ketchup
- ¼ cup mustard (I used yellow, if using stoneground or dijon, consider using slightly less)
- ¼ cup molasses (use mild/light/medium, not dark/robust/blackstrap)
- ¼ cup olive oil

- ¼ cup apple cider vinegar
- 2 tablespoons Worcestershire sauce (omit if keeping vegan, or substitute with Bragg's Liquid Aminos or soy sauce)

Directions

1. Rinse and sort dry beans in a colander over the sink.
2. Add beans to a large pot and cover with 8 cups water and let soak overnight (about 8 hours). OR to save time.
3. Use the 1 hour rapid soak method. Bring beans and 8 cups water to a boil. Allow beans to boil rapidly for 3 minutes, uncovered. Shut the heat off, cover the pot, and let stand for 1 hour.
4. In either the overnight soak method or the 1 hour rapid soak method, drain soaking water and rinse beans well under running water in a colander over the sink.
5. Return beans to pot, cover with 6 cups water, and allow to simmer on low heat for about 45 minutes, or until quite tender; cooked about 80% of the way. They'll be transferred to a slow cooker where they'll cook for 12+ hours so you don't want them or need them to be totally done, but they shouldn't be overly hard either (taste a few beans, you'll know when you bite into them)
6. While beans are simmering, combine all remaining ingredients in the slow cooker, and whisk to combine until smooth.

7. After beans are done simmering, drain them, add them to the slow cooker, and stir.

8. Cover and cook on low heat for about 12 hours (start checking at about 8 hours), or until beans are tender, the sauce has thickened and reduced dramatically, the flavor is concentrated and robust, and the smell in your house is intoxicating. If after 12 hours your sauce is still liquidy or on the soupy side, remove the lid, increase the heat to the highest setting, and cook uncovered until thickened to desired level (this took 4 hours for me; 12 hours covered on low and 4 hours uncovered on high, for 16 hours total). Note – Because slow-cookers and temperatures vary greatly, you can tinker with the temperature settings as you see fit. You could possibly cook on medium for 10 to 12 hours, or cook on high for 8 to 10 hours, or do a combination of settings until your sauce has thickened and beans are tender.

9. Serve immediately. Beans will keep airtight in the refrigerator for up to 1 week, and taste better on days 2 and 3 as the flavor marry even more. I would anticipate finished beans could be frozen for up to 6 months, however I have not tested it. Take care all ingredients used are suitable for your dietary needs if keeping vegan and gluten-free, reading labels and selecting specific brands that meet your needs.

Slow Cooker Chipotle Tacos

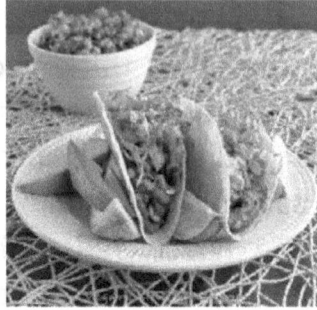

Serves: 4

Cook Time: 4 hours
Ingredients

- 30 ounces pinto beans 2 cans, 15 ounce each, drained
- 1 cup corn canned, frozen or fresh
- 3 ounces chipotle pepper in adobo sauce, chopped
- 6 ounces tomato paste 1 can
- ¾ cup Chili Sauce
- 1 tablespoon Unsweetened Cocoa Powder
- 1 teaspoon Ground Cumin
- ½ teaspoon Ground Cinnamon
- 8 taco shells hard white corn or your favorite, hard or soft
- favorite toppings = lettuce, avocado, lime

Directions

1. Well, here we go. I am all about 'easy' cooking.
2. Put everything in the crockpot.
3. Cook on low 3 to 4 hours or on high 1-½ to 2 hours.
4. Spread quite a bit on your favorite taco shells, hard or soft.
5. Top with lettuce (I used sliced romaine).
6. You can also add fresh tomatoes, and avocado. Lime is a nice touch too.
7. Serve with some beans and rice if you like.

Slow Cooker Vegan Butternut Squash Soup

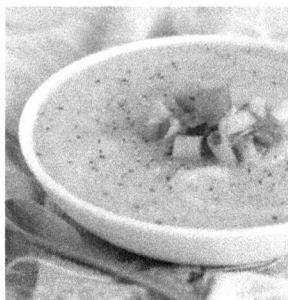

Serves: 4

Cook Time: 6 hours
Ingredients

- 1 medium butternut squash (1 lb of peeled and cubed butternut squash)

- 1 medium onion, diced
- ½ lb carrots, peeled and cut into chunks
- 1 granny smith apple, peeled and sliced
- 3 cups vegetable broth
- 1 bay leaf
- 1 tsp salt
- 1 tsp pepper
- ¼ tsp dried ground sage
- 1 (13.5 oz) can coconut milk
- Salt and pepper to taste

Directions

1. Combine squash, onion, carrots, apple, broth and bay leaf in slow cooker.
2. Cover and cook on LOW for about 6 hours, or until veggies are soft.
3. Remove bay leaf and discard. Transfer contents of slow cooker to a blender and blend until smooth (or you can use an immersion blender).
4. When smooth, pour back into the slow cooker and add in salt, pepper, sage and coconut milk. Stir. Taste and then add more salt and pepper to taste. (I probably added in an additional ½ tsp of salt)
5. Serve and enjoy with croutons or crusty bread.

Italian Eggplant Casserole With Cashew-Tofu Ricotta

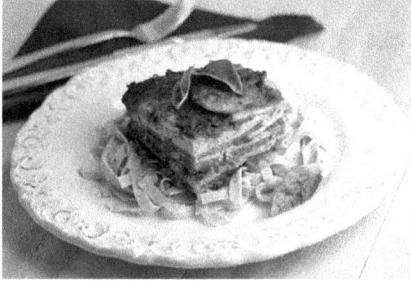

Serves: 4

Cook Time: 3 hours
Ingredients

The Cashew-Tofu Ricotta:

- ½ cup (68gm) cashews (I used 2oz, or 56gm)
- ½ cup (48gm) nutritional yeast
- 3 cloves of garlic
- 1 15oz package of firm tofu
- ½ cup unsweetened nondairy milk
- 2 teaspoons lemon juice (my addition)
- ½ teaspoon salt
- Freshly ground black pepper, to taste

Remaining Ingredients:

- 1 large eggplant (about 1 ¼lb), thinly sliced

- 1 jar (25oz, or 700gm) marinara sauce, store-bought or homemade
- Cooked pasta, for serving

Directions

The Night Before:

1. Make the ricotta by blending all of the ingredients in a food processor or blender until smooth. Store in a covered container in the refrigerator.

In the Morning:

1. Oil the crock of your slow cooker (or spray lightly with cooking spray.) Pour in 1/3 of the marinara sauce. Top with half of the eggplant slices, half of the ricotta, and another 1/3 of the sauce. Repeat the layers once more, then top with the remaining sauce. (I sliced my eggplant thin enough that I ended up with three layers each of eggplant and ricotta, alternated with sauce.) Cover and cook on low for 6-8 hours. Serve with pasta.

2. If your slow cooker does not run hot and the dish seems water, remove the lid and turn the slow cooker to high. The liquid should evaporate in 30-60 minutes.

Teriyaki Tofu With Kale And Rice

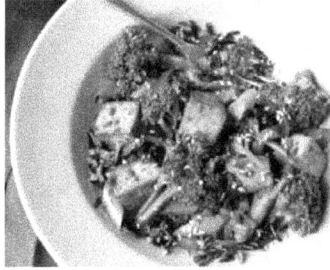

Serves: 4

Cook Time: 3 hours
Ingredients

- 2-1 pound packages firm or extra firm tofu
- 1 cup pineapple juice
- ½ cup vegetable broth
- ½ cup tamari or good soy sauce
- ¼ cup mirin
- ¼ cup unseasoned rice vinegar
- 2 tbsp brown sugar
- 1 tbsp sesame oil
- 1 tbsp grated ginger (more or less, according to taste)
- 3-4 cloves of garlic, grated or very finely minced

- 6 pineapple rings, fresh or canned
- rice, for serving
- fresh, shredded kale, for serving

Directions

1. Drain the tofu, and cut each block into 6 rectangular slices. Press the tofu, to remove the excess water. Cut the pressed tofu pieces in half, to make squares. Then cut the squares on the diagonal, to make triangles. Set aside.

2. In a medium sized bowl, whisk together the juice, broth, tamari, mirin, vinegar, sugar, oil, ginger, and garlic.

3. Place the pineapple in a large casserole dish. Top with the tofu triangles. Then pour the sauce over the tofu.

4. Bake, uncovered, for 2-3 hours at 325 degrees. You can baste the tofu a couple times during baking, if you wish.

5. Serve over a bed of rice and kale.

Vegan Jambalaya

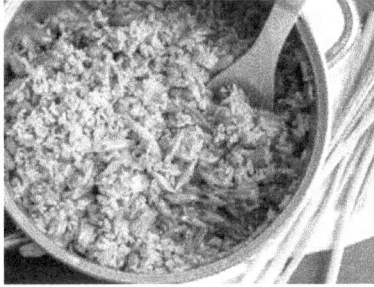

Serves: 4

Cook Time: 4 hours
Ingredients

- 6 oz soy chorizo (optional)
- 1 green bell pepper, diced
- 1 cup okra, ½" inch rounds
- ½ onion, diced
- 3 celery ribs (about 1½ cups)
- 2 cloves garlic, minced
- 1 16-oz can of Rotel (diced tomatoes & green chilis)
- 1½ cups vegetable broth
- ½ tsp paprika
- ¼ tsp salt
- ¼ tsp ground black pepper
- ¼ tsp cayenne pepper

- 3 cups cooked cilantro rice

Directions

1. Begin by cooking the chorizo in a skillet on medium-high heat. Let simmer until brown, then place in the crockpot.

2. Next, add the diced bell pepper, onion, celery, garlic and okra to the slow cooker. Then, pour in the diced tomatoes and vegetable broth.

3. Add the seasoning and give the vegetables a nice stir.

4. Cook on low for 4-6 hours or on high for about 2 hours.

5. About 30 minutes before the jambalaya will be served, mix the cooked rice into the slow cooker and laissez les bons temps rouler!

2. Tasty Recipes

Ratatouille

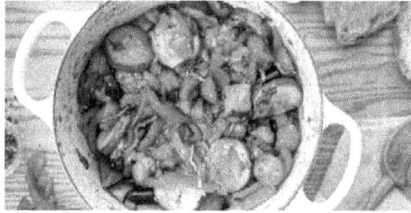

Serves: 4

Cook Time: 9 hours
Ingredients

- 2 large onions, cut in half and sliced
- 1 large eggplant, sliced, cut in 2 inch pieces
- 4 small zucchini, sliced
- 2 garlic cloves, minced
- 2 large green bell peppers, de-seeded and cut into thin strips
- 2 large tomatoes, cut into ½ inch wedges
- 1 (6 ounce) can tomato paste
- 1 teaspoon dried basil
- ½ teaspoon oregano
- 1 teaspoon sugar
- 2 teaspoons salt

- ½ teaspoon black pepper
- 2 tablespoons fresh parsley, chopped
- ¼ cup olive oil
- red pepper flakes, to spice it up

Directions

1. Layer half the vegetables in a large crock pot in the following order: onion, eggplant, zucchini, garlic, green peppers, tomatoes.
2. Next sprinkle half the basil, oregano, sugar, parsley, salt and pepper on the veggies.
3. Dot with half of the tomato paste.
4. Repeat layering process with remaining vegetables, spices and tomato paste.
5. Drizzle with olive oil.
6. Cover and cook on LOW for 7 to 9 hours.
7. Place in serving bowl and sprinkle with freshly grated Parmesan cheese.
8. Refrigerate to store.

Pinto Beans And Rice

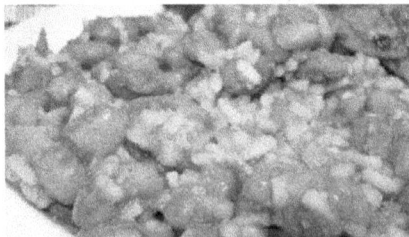

Serves: 4

Cook Time: 3 hours

Ingredients

- 1 (1 lb) bag dried pinto bean
- ⅓ cup picante sauce
- 2 ½ teaspoons salt
- ½ teaspoon pepper
- 1 teaspoon garlic powder
- 1 tablespoon garlic, minced (kind in jar is okay)
- 1 tablespoon chili powder
- ½ teaspoon cumin
- ½ teaspoon oregano
- 3 bay leaves
- 1 cup cooked white rice

Directions

1. Rinse beans in colander.
2. Put in a crock pot (or large pot).
3. Cover with water, plus about 2 inches over top of beans.
4. Add all ingredients, except rice.
5. Cook on high in crock pot about 3 hours til tender. (Crockpots vary greatly on cooking times. It could take much longer in yours, so the first time allow longer to cook and then you will know how long cooking time will be in the future.).

6. (Add water if necessary) May also cook on low overnight.
7. Add rice and cook until rice is warm.
8. Serve with cornbread.

Lentil-Veggie Soup

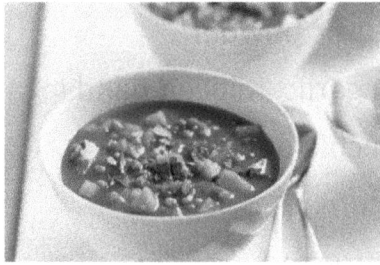

Serves: 4

Cook Time: 12 hours
Ingredients

- 1 cup dry lentils
- 1 ½ cups carrots, chopped
- 1 ½ cups celery, chopped
- 1 ½ cups onions, chopped
- 3 garlic cloves, minced
- 1 teaspoon dried basil
- 1 teaspoon dried oregano
- ½ teaspoon dried thyme

- 1 tablespoon dried parsley
- 2 bay leaves
- 3 ½ cups vegetable broth (2 cans)
- 1 ½ cups water
- 1 (14 ½ ounce) can diced tomatoes
- fresh ground black pepper, to taste

Directions

1. Rinse lentils.
2. Place all ingredients except the pepper into a 4-6 quart slow cooker.
3. Cover and cook on low for at least 12 hours, or high for at least 5 hours.
4. Season with pepper and remove the bay leaves before serving.

Spicy Black Beans And Rice With Mangoes

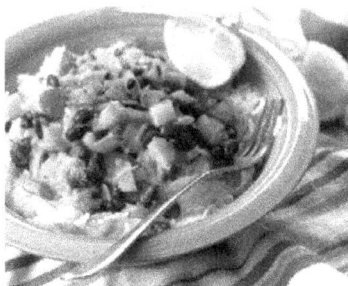

Serves: 4

Cook Time: 6 hours

Ingredients

- 1 tablespoon olive oil
- 1 small onion, finely chopped
- ½ red bell pepper, seeded and chopped
- 2 garlic cloves, minced
- 1 jalapeno, seeded and minced (any hot chile pepper okay)
- 1 teaspoon fresh ginger, peeled and minced
- ½ teaspoon ground cumin
- ½ teaspoon ground allspice
- ½ teaspoon dried oregano
- 2 (15 ½ ounce) cans black beans, drained and rinsed
- 1 cup water
- ½ teaspoon light brown sugar
- ½ teaspoon salt
- ¼ teaspoon black pepper, freshly ground
- 3 cups cooked long-grain brown rice (white rice okay)
- 2 mangoes, ripe, medium sized, peeled and flesh diced

Directions

1. Heat oil in large skillet over medium heat.
2. Add onion, bell pepper, garlic and jalapeno, cover, and cook 5 minutes until softened.
3. Add in seasonings, mix well and cook for 1 minute.

4. Transfer mixture into a 3 ½ to 4 quart slow cooker.

5. Add bean, water, brown sugar, salt and pepper.

6. Stir well.

7. Cover and cook on low for 6 to 8 hours.

8. Add the cooked rice and the mangoes.

9. Allow to cook another 10 minutes.

10. Serve and enjoy.

Spicy Chickpeas

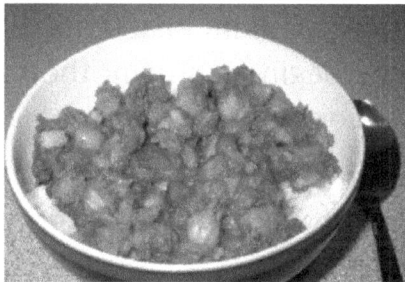

Serves: 4

Cook Time: 8 hours
Ingredients

- 1 tablespoon vegetable oil

- 2 onions, peeled and finely chopped

- 4 garlic cloves, finely chopped

- 2 tablespoons minced fresh gingerroot

- 2 teaspoons ground coriander

- 1 teaspoon cumin seed
- 1 teaspoon salt
- ½ teaspoon fresh ground black pepper
- ½ teaspoon cayenne pepper (reduce if that's too spicy for your tastes)
- 2 teaspoons balsamic vinegar
- 2 cups coarsely chopped tomatoes (, canned or fresh)
- 2 (19 ounce) cans chickpeas, rinsed and drained

Directions

1. In a skillet over medium heat, cook onions, stirring, just until they begin to brown; then add garlic and all spices and cook, stirring, for 1 minute.
2. Add vinegar and tomatoes and bring to a boil, then place mixture in your slow cooker; add chickpeas and combine well.
3. Cover and cook on Low for 6 to 8 hours or on High for 3 to 4 hours, or until the mixture is hot and bubbling.
4. Serve with hot naan or pita bread.

Yummy And Super Easy Oatmeal

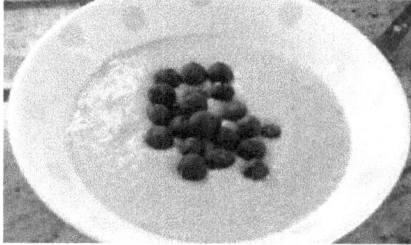

Serves: 4

Cook Time: 10 hours
Ingredients

- 2 cups old fashioned oats (I get this in bulk from my food co-op, if you used the quick cooking ones, it might be even creamier)
- 6 cups water, I think you need more than usual because of the long cooking time
- cinnamon (optional)
- dried fruits (optional)
- spices (optional)

Directions

1. Put the oats and the water, along with anything else you want to add to the mix in the crock pot, turn on to low, and go to bed thinking about what a great breakfast you›re going to have!

2. I scoop it out of the crock pot and eat it with maple syrup, or blueberry syrup, or pourable fruit, and soy milk--yum!
3. To reheat leftovers, I usually add a little water, and stir it a couple of times while microwaving until it›s hot.
4. You can add other flavorings as you like, such as dried fruits, other sweet spices, diced apples, etc.
5. I usually put raisins on after it›s cooked because I like them chewy.
6. I›ve been meaning to try dried cranberries.

Slow Cooker Enchilada Quinoa

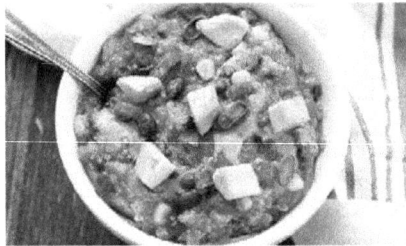

Serves: 4

Cook Time: 4 hours
Ingredients

- 1 15-ounce can black beans, drained and rinsed
- 1 15-ounce can yellow corn, drained and rinsed

- 2 15-ounce cans of mild or medium red enchilada sauce, divided
- 1 15-ounce can of diced fire roasted tomatoes and green chiles
- 1 cup un-cooked quinoa + ½ cup water
- 4 ounces cream cheese (light or fat free is okay)
- salt and pepper to taste (I used about 1 teaspoon salt and ¼ teaspoon black pepper)
- 1 cup shredded Mexican style cheese
- optional: chopped cilantro, diced tomatoes, diced avocado, sour cream

Directions

1. Add beans, corn, 1 can of enchilada sauce, diced tomatoes and chiles, quinoa, water, cream cheese, and salt and pepper to the slow cooker. Stir everything together.
2. Pour remaining can of enchilada sauce on top, then sprinkle with shredded cheese. Cover and cook 4-5 hours on high or 5-7 hours on low.
3. Uncover, top with tomatoes, avocados, sour cream, and chopped cilantro and serve.

Chickpea & Sweet Potato Chili

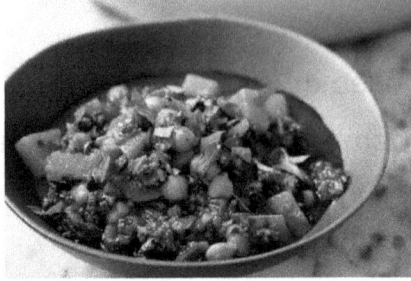

Serves: 4

Cook Time: 8 hours
Ingredients

Chili

- 28 oz can of diced tomatoes
- 13.5 oz can of tomato sauce (400mL)
- 4 tablespoons adobo sauce (for less spicy version) + 1 chopped chipotle pepper (for spicy)
- 2 tablespoons chili powder
- 1 tsp ground cumin
- 1 tsp salt
- ½ cup stock
- 1 large sweet potato, peeled and cut into 1.5-2 inch cubes (roughly 5 cups/700g)
- 4 cloves garlic, minced
- 2 medium onions, diced
- 2 carrots, peeled and diced

- 2 19 oz cans of chickpeas, drained and rinsed

After cooking

- Juice of half a lime
- To Serve (Optional)
- Avocado
- Cilantro leaves
- Sour cream or Greek yogurt
- Tortilla chips

Directions

1. Add all ingredients to the base of a 5 quart slow cooker. Mix with a spatula until completely combined.
2. At this point, the slow cooker insert may be refrigerated overnight, until ready to cook.
3. Cook on lowest setting for 8-10 hours.
4. Before serving, *gently* stir in the lime juice.
5. Serve with avocado, cilantro, yogurt/sour cream, and tortilla chips.

Quinoa And Black Bean Stuffed Peppers

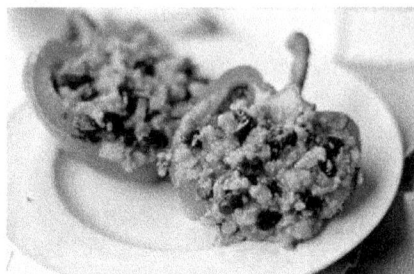

Serves: 4

Cook Time: 4 hours
Ingredients

- 6 bell peppers
- 1 cup uncooked quinoa, rinsed
- 1 14 ounce can black beans, rinsed and drained
- 1 14 ounce can refried beans
- 1 ½ cups red enchilada sauce
- 1 teaspoon cumin
- 1 teaspoon chili powder
- 1 teaspoon onion powder
- ½ teaspoon garlic salt
- 1 ½ cups shredded Pepperjack cheese
- Toppings! Cilantro, avocado, sour cream, etc.

Directions

1. Cut the tops off of the peppers and scrape out the ribs and seeds.

2. In a large bowl, combine the quinoa, beans, enchilada sauce, spices, and 1 cup of the cheese. Fill each pepper with the quinoa mixture.

3. Pour ½ cup water into the bottom of a crockpot. Place the peppers in the crockpot so they're sitting in the water. Cover and cook on low for 6 hours or high for 3 hours. Remove lid, distribute remaining cheese over the tops of the peppers, and cover again for a few minutes to melt the cheese.

4. Serve topped with anything you like! These are also great with chips and guacamole, believe it or not.

Slow Cooker White Bean Stew

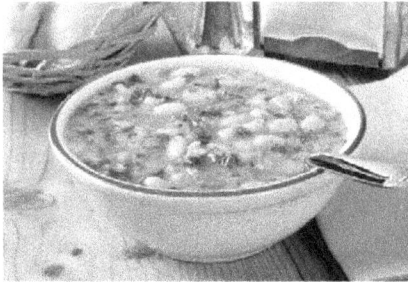

Serves: 4

Cook Time: 4 hours

Ingredients

- 2 pounds white beans
- 2 large carrots, peeled and diced
- 3 large celery stalks, diced
- 1 onion, diced
- 3 cloves garlic, minced or chopped
- 1 bay leaf
- 1 tsp. each: dried rosemary, thyme, oregano
- 10-12 cups water
- 2 Tbsp. salt
- Ground black pepper, to taste
- 1 large can (28 ounces) diced tomatoes
- 5-6 cups (or more) roughly chopped leafy greens (spinach, chard, kale)
- Rice, polenta, or bread for serving

Directions

1. Sort through and rinse beans several times in cool water. Add to the slow cooker along with the diced carrots, celery, onions, garlic, bay leaf and dried herbs. Add the water. (Use less for a thicker stew, more for more of a soup.) Cover and cook on HIGH for 3-4 hours, or LOW for 8-10 hours. Remove lid from slow cooker and add the salt and pepper, and diced tomatoes. Let cook for another 1-1½ hours, or until beans are very soft. (If they are already soft after the initial cooking time, different kinds of beans may vary in cooking time, then add the

tomatoes and greens and serve immediately.) Before serving, stir in the chopped greens.

2. Serve over hot cooked rice, polenta, or with bread.

3. Makes a lot--enough for at least 10-12 servings. Freeze half for later or invite friends over.

Curried Vegetable & Chickpea Stew

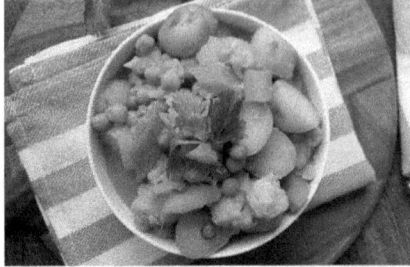

Serves: 4

Cook Time: 4 hours
Ingredients

- 1 teaspoon olive oil
- 1 large onion, diced
- 1 tablespoon kosher salt, divided
- 2 medium red or yellow potatoes, diced
- 1 tablespoon curry powder
- 1 tablespoon packed brown sugar
- 1 tablespoon peeled and grated fresh ginger
- 3 cloves garlic, minced
- ⅛ teaspoon cayenne pepper (optional)
- 2 cups low-sodium vegetable broth, divided
- 2 (15-ounce) cans chickpeas, drained and rinsed
- 1 medium green bell pepper, diced

- 1 medium red bell pepper, diced
- 1 medium head cauliflower, cut into bite-sized florets
- 1 (28-ounce) can diced tomatoes with their juices
- ¼ teaspoon freshly ground black pepper
- 1 (10-ounce) bag baby spinach
- 1 cup coconut milk

Directions

1. Heat the oil in a large frying pan over medium heat until shimmering. Add the onion, season with 1 teaspoon of the salt, and sauté until translucent, about 5 minutes. Add the potatoes and 1 teaspoon of the salt, and sauté until just translucent around the edges.

2. Stir in the curry, brown sugar, ginger, garlic, and cayenne if using and cook until fragrant, about 30 seconds. Pour in ¼ cup of the broth and scrape up any browned bits from the bottom of the pan. Transfer this onion-potato mixture into the bowl of a 6-quart or larger slow cooker. (Halve this recipe for a smaller slow cooker.)

3. Add the remaining 1 ¾ cups broth, chickpeas, bell peppers, cauliflower, tomatoes with their juices, pepper, and remaining 1 teaspoon salt. Stir to combine. The liquid should come about halfway up the sides of the bowl; add more broth as needed. Cover and cook for on the HIGH setting for 4 hours.

4. Stir in the spinach and coconut milk. Cover and let sit for a few more minutes to allow the spinach to wilt. Taste and season with salt and other seasonings as needed. Serve on its own, or over couscous, Israeli couscous, or orzo pasta.

Spaghetti Squash Thai Noodle Bowl

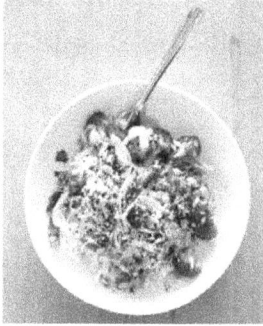

Serves: 4

Cook Time: 8 hours
Ingredients

- 1 Small Spaghetti Squash (About 4-5 lbs.)
- 2 C. Water
- 2 C. Broccoli, Steamed
- ½ Batch Prepared Skinny Thai Peanut Dressing (I used Lime Juice instead of ½ of the Vinegar for mine.)
- 1 Tbsp. Sesame Seeds
- Optional/Suggested Toppings:
- Chopped Peanuts
- Sriracha

Directions

1. Pierce your spaghetti squash all over with a fork (similarly to how you would with a potato before baking.)

2. Place the squash and 2 c. of water into a slow cooker. Secure the lid and cook for 8-9 hours on low.

3. The squash will turn brownish and kind of dingy while cooking, but don›t let that scare you. The insides are perfectly perfect!

4. Once done, remove the squash from the crock pot and set aside to cool for 20-30 minutes. Discard the water.

5. After the squash has cooled, cut it in half and scoop out the seeds and pulp.

6. It should all come out pretty easily. Mine even separated from the meat of the squash on it›s own.

7. Discard or use for something else if you want.

8. With the pulp removed, use a fork to shred the insides into spaghetti like noodles.

9. Feel free to get all the way down to the flesh of the squash.

10. Place the ‹noodles› into a bowl and top each with 1 c. of broccoli, 3 tbsp. dressing, ½ tbsp. sesame seeds, and peanuts if desired. Enjoy!

3. Fast And Easy Recipes

Slow Cooker Lentil Bolognese

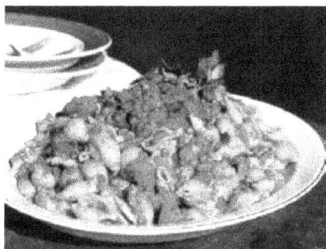

Serves: 4

Cook Time: 5 hours
Ingredients

- 1 large sweet onion, diced
- 2 carrots, diced
- 3 celery stalks, diced
- 8 garlic cloves, minced
- Salt & pepper
- 1 16-ounce bag dried lentils, rinsed and picked through
- 2 28-ounce cans crushed tomatoes
- 5 cups water
- 3 tablespoons bouillon powder (about 8 cubes)
- 1 bay leaf
- 2 tablespoons dried basil

- 2 teaspoons dried parsley
- 1 teaspoon coarse salt
- ½ - 1 teaspoon crushed red pepper flakes

Directions

1. In a large slow cooker, mix together the onion, carrot, celery and garlic. Season liberally with salt and pepper.
2. Add the remaining ingredients and stir to combine.
3. Cook on low for 4 - 5 hours, or until lentils have softened and sauce is thick.
4. Adjust seasoning with salt & pepper to taste.

Slow Cooker Burrito Bowls

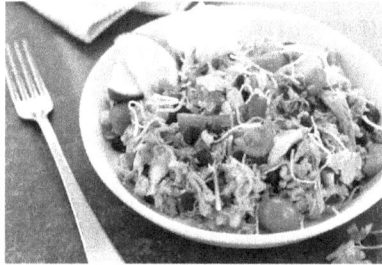

Serves: 4

Cook Time: 3 hours
Ingredients

- 1 onion, diced or thinly sliced
- 1 bell pepper (I used yellow), diced
- 1 mild red chilli, finely chopped
- 400 g tin black beans, drained (240g, or ~ 1 ¼ cups, when drained)
- 215 g uncooked brown rice (~ 1 cup)
- 400 g tin chopped tomatoes (~ 1 ½ cups)
- 150 ml water (~ ½ cup)
- 1 tbsp chipotle hot sauce (or other favourite hot sauce)
- 1 tsp smoked paprika
- ½ tsp ground cumin
- Salt

- Black pepper
- To serve, your choice of: grated cheese, fresh coriander (cilantro), chopped spring onions, sliced avocado, sour cream, guacamole, etc.

Directions

1. Add all the burrito bowl ingredients (not toppings) to a slow cooker - mine is 4.7 litres / 4 quarts. Mix well.
2. Cook on low for around 3 hours, or until the rice is cooked.
3. Serve hot with your choice of toppings.

Slow Cooker Lentil And Quinoa Chili

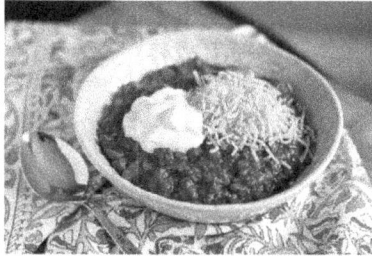

Serves: 4

Cook Time: 4 hours
Ingredients

- 1 onion, chopped
- 3 garlic cloves, minced
- 1 celery stalk, chopped
- 2 bell peppers, chopped
- 1 15 oz can diced tomatoes
- 4 cups vegetable broth
- 1 can water (I use the can of diced tomatoes to grab all the leftover flavor)
- 1 cup dried lentils
- 1 15 oz can Bush's Pinto Beans
- 2 tablespoons chili powder
- 2 teaspoons cumin

119

- 1 tablespoon oregano
- ½ cup uncooked quinoa

Directions

1. Place all ingredients into slow cooker. Cook on low heat for 8 hours.

Slow Cooker Veggie Pot Pie

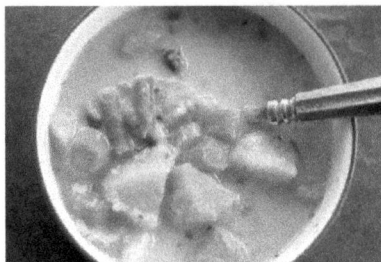

Serves: 4

Cook Time: 6 hours
Ingredients

- 6-7 cups veggies chopped into bite sized pieces as needed (I used: brussels sprouts, frozen corn kernels, frozen peas, diced potatoes, baby carrots, and pre-sliced mushrooms)
- diced onion (½ cup)
- minced garlic (4 cloves)
- fresh thyme (5-6 sprigs, leaves removed and chopped)

- ¼ cup flour
- 2 cups chicken broth
- ¼ cup cornstarch
- ¼ cup heavy cream
- salt and pepper to taste
- 1 frozen puff pastry sheet, thawed
- 2 tablespoons butter

Directions

1. Clean and chop veggies as needed and add to slow cooker along with onion and garlic
2. Toss with flour to coat well
3. Slowly stir in broth until well blended with flour
4. Cover and cook on high for 3-4 hours or low for 6-8
5. Whisk cornstarch with ¼ cup water until smooth then stir into the veggie mixure
6. Stir in cream, cover, and return slow cooker to high heat for about 15 minutes or until mixture thickens slightly
7. Transfer to a 9x13 baking dish and top with thawed puff pastry sheet (cut to fit if necessary)
8. Melt 2 tablespoons of butter and brush over top of pastry
9. Bake at 400 degrees for about 10 minutes or until pastry is golden and fluffy

Slow Cooker Butternut Squash Macaroni

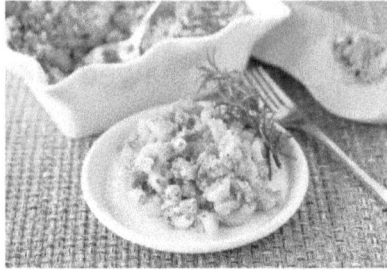

Serves: 4

Cook Time: 7 hours
Ingredients

FOR THE MORNING

- 1 ½ cups (210 g) cubed butternut squash or other winter squash
- ½ cup (90 g) chopped tomatoes
- 1 ½ cups (355 ml) water
- 2 cloves garlic, minced
- Three 3-inch (7.5 cm) sprigs fresh thyme or 1 ½ teaspoons (1.5 g) dried thyme
- One 2-inch (5 cm) sprig fresh rosemary or ½ teaspoon dried rosemary

FOR THE EVENING

- ¼ cup (24 g) nutritional yeast flakes
- ½ to 1 cup (120 to 235 ml) unsweetened nondairy milk
- 1 ½ cups (158 g) uncooked whole-wheat macaroni (*use gluten-free)
- Salt and pepper, to taste

Directions

1. In the morning: Add the morning ingredients to the slow cooker. Cook on low for 7 to 9 hours.
2. Thirty to 45 minutes before serving: Purée the contents of the slow cooker in a blender with the nutritional yeast and ½ cup (120 ml) of the nondairy milk. Add the mixture back into the slow cooker and turn it up to high. Stir in the macaroni, cover, and cook for 20 minutes.
3. Stir well and add more milk if the sauce is getting too thick. Cook for 15 to 25 minutes more or until the pasta is al dente. Add salt and pepper to taste.
4. Make sure to check on the pasta every 10 minutes or so until you get good at gauging how fast it will cook in your slow cooker. It cooks faster in the smaller slow cooker.

Slow Cooker Coconut Quinoa Curry

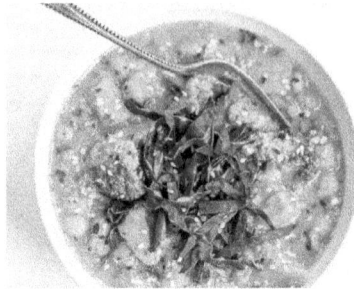

Serves: 4

Cook Time: 4 hours
Ingredients

- 1 medium sweet potato, peeled + chopped (about 3 cups)
- 1 large broccoli crown, cut into florets (about 2 cups)
- ½ white onion, diced (about 1 cup)
- 1 (15 oz) can organic chickpeas, drained and rinsed
- 1 (28 oz) can diced tomatoes
- 2 (14.5 oz) cans coconut milk (either full fat or lite)
- ¼ cup quinoa
- 2 garlic cloves, minced (about 1 tablespoon)
- 1 tablespoon freshly grated ginger
- 1 tablespoon freshly grated turmeric (or 1 teaspoon ground)

- 2 teaspoon wheat free tamari sauce
- 1 teaspoon miso (or additional tamari)
- ½ – 1 teaspoon chili flakes

Directions

1. Add all ingredients to a slow cooker, starting with 1 cup of water. Stir until everything is fully incorporated.
2. Turn the slow cooker to high and cook for 3 – 4 hours until sweet potato cooks through and the curry has thickened.

Slow Cooker Split Pea Soup

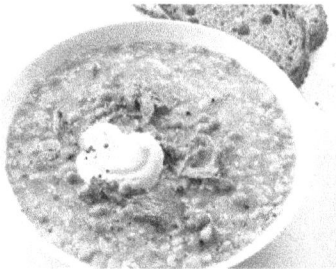

Serves: 4

Cook Time: 7 hours

Ingredients

- 1 16-oz package (1 lb) dried green split peas, rinsed
- 1 large leek (light green and white portion only), chopped and thoroughly cleaned

- 3 celery ribs, diced
- 2 large carrots, diced
- 1 garlic clove, minced
- ¼ cup chopped fresh parsley
- 6 cups vegetable broth
- ½ t ground black pepper
- 1 t salt, or to taste
- 1 bay leaf

Directions

1. Pour all of the ingredients in a slow cooker and stir to combine.
2. Cover a cook on low for 7 to 8 hours or high 3 to 4 hours.
3. Remove and discard bay leaf before serving. Enjoy!

Slow Cooker Masala Lentils

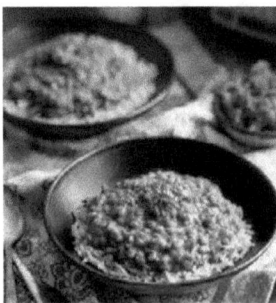

Serves: 4

Cook Time: 6 hours

Ingredients

- 1 yellow onion, chopped
- 3 cloves garlic, minced
- 1 tablespoon minced fresh ginger, or 1 teaspoon ground ginger powder
- 2¼ cups brown, green or pardina lentils
- 4 cups vegetable broth
- 1 15-ounce can diced or stewed tomatoes, with their juices
- ¼ cup tomato paste
- 2 teaspoons tamarind paste (optional, adds a hint of tartness)
- 1 teaspoon maple syrup
- ¾ teaspoon salt
- 1½ teaspoon garam masala
- A few shakes black pepper
- 1 cup light coconut milk
- For serving: Rice, quinoa, or another whole grain | Fresh herbs

Directions

1. Place all ingredients except for the coconut milk in your slow cooker. Stir. Cook on high heat for 3-4 hours or on low heat for 6 hours. In the last hour or two of cooking, respectively, check to see if the lentils need more liquid, and add extra broth or

water. You can adjust this based on how thick you›d like the finished lentils to be, keeping in mind that you›ll be adding more liquid in the form of the coconut milk.

2. When the lentils are ready, stir in the co

Vegan Mexican Bowl

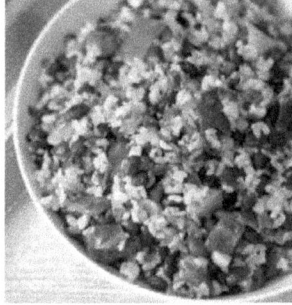

Serves: 4

Cook Time: 3 hours
Ingredients

Slow Cooker Ingredients:

- 1 cup long-grain brown rice (I used Uncle Ben's Brown Rice)
- 2 cups vegetable stock (I used a can of vegetable broth and a little water to make 2 cups)
- 1 cup finely chopped onion

- 1 red bell pepper, chopped small
- 1 green bell pepper, chopped small
- 1 can (4 oz.) diced green chiles plus juice (Anaheim chiles, not jalapenos)
- 2 cans (15 oz.) black beans, rinsed well and drained
- salt to taste

Salsa Ingredients:

- ½ cup diced tomato
- 1 large Poblano pepper, very finely diced
- ½ cup thinly sliced green onion
- ½ cup finely chopped fresh cilantro
- 1 large avocado (or 2 small avocadoes) cut into cubes about 1 inch
- 1 T + 2 T fresh lime juice
- 2 T extra-virgin olive oil
- ½ tsp. ground cumin (or more, to taste)
- salt to taste

Directions

1. Combine the rice, vegetable stock, and finely chopped onion in the slow cooker and cook on high for 1 ½ hours, or until rice is just starting to get tender. While rice cooks, chop the red and green bell pepper, and open the diced green chiles. Drain the black beans into a colander placed in the sink and rinse well with cold water until no more foam appears; then let beans drain well.

2. After 1 ½ hours, add the chopped red bell pepper, chopped green bell pepper, diced green chiles with juice, and drained black beans to the slow cooker and gently combine with the rice. Add salt to taste and then cook on high for about 30 minutes more.

3. While the rice mixture finishes cooking, chop the tomato, cilantro, and Poblano pepper and thinly slice the green onion. Cut the avocado into cubes about 1 inch across and toss in a bowl with 1 T of lime juice. (Use a bowl that will hold all the salsa ingredients. Add the chopped tomato, chopped cilantro, finely chopped Poblano, sliced green onion, other 2 T lime juice, 2 T olive oil, ground cumin, and salt to taste, and gently combine.

4. The slow cooker mixture is ready when the rice is tender (and preferably the peppers are barely cooked, with still quite a bit of crunch.) Serve hot or warm, with a generous scoop of the Poblano-Avocado Salsa on top. You could add other toppings such as desired.

Black Bean Pumpkin Chili

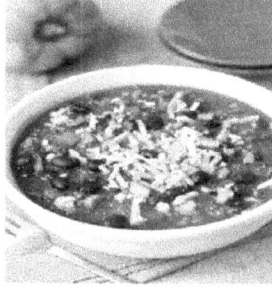

Serves: 4

Cook Time: 8 hours
Ingredients

- 3 (15-ounce) cans black beans, drained
- 2 (14.5-ounce)cans plain diced tomatoes
- 1 cup pureed pumpkin (not pumpkin pie mix)
- 2 cups diced yellow onion (about 1 medium onion)
- 1 medium yellow bell pepper, diced
- 1 tablespoon chili powder
- 1 teaspoon cinnamon
- 1 teaspoon cumin
- ¼ teaspoon nutmeg
- ⅛ teaspoon ground cloves
- ½ teaspoon kosher salt
- ½ teaspoon coarse ground black pepper

- Assorted toppings of your choice like avocado, cherry tomatoes, chopped scallions or onion, cilantro, Tapatio sauce (if you want to add some heat), or, if not vegan, shredded cheddar or jack cheese and sour cream.

Directions

1. Add all ingredients to a 4-quart or larger slow cooker. Stir.
2. Cook on low for 8 – 10 hours.
3. Serve with assorted toppings.

Cauliflower Bolognese With Zucchini Noodles

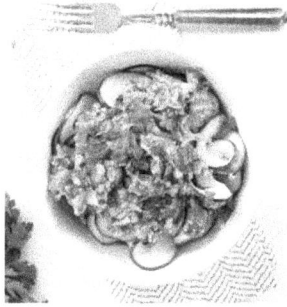

Serves: 4

Cook Time: 3.5 hours
Ingredients

For the bolognese:
- 1 head of cauliflower, cut up into florets
- ¾ cup diced red onion
- 2 small garlic cloves, minced
- 2 tsp dried oregano flakes
- 1 tsp dried basil flakes
- 2 14oz cans diced tomatoes, no salt added
- ½ cup vegetable broth, low-sodium
- ¼ tsp red pepper flakes
- salt and pepper, to taste

For the pasta:
- 5 large zucchinis, Blade A

Directions

1. Place all of the ingredients for the bolognese into a crockpot. Place the crockpot on high and let cook for 3.5 hours.

2. When done, smash the cauliflower with a potato masher or fork until the florets break up to create a "bolognese."

3. Spoon the bolognese over bowls of zucchini noodles.

Vindaloo Vegetables

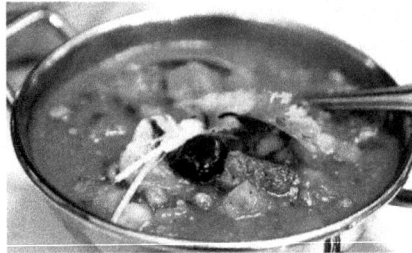

Serves: 4

Cook Time: 35 minutes
Ingredients

- 3 cloves garlic peeled
- 1 tablespoon ginger peeled and chopped
- 1 pitted date coarsely chopped

- 1 ½ teaspoon ground coriander
- 1 ¼ teaspoon ground cumin
- ½ teaspoon dry mustard
- ½ teaspoon cayenne pepper or to taste
- ½ teaspoon turmeric
- ¼ teaspoon cardamom
- 1 tablespoon white wine vinegar
- 1 large yellow onion chopped
- 2 small carrots thinly sliced
- 4 cups small cauliflower florets
- 1 ½ cups cooked kidney beans or one 15.5 ounce can, rinsed and drained
- 6 ounces tomato paste (one small can)
- 2 small zucchini cut into ¼-inch-thick slices
- 1 small green or red bell pepper seeded and diced
- Salt and freshly ground black pepper to taste
- 1 cup frozen green peas thawed

Directions

1. In a blender or food processor, combine the garlic, ginger, date, coriander and other spices, vinegar, and ½ cup water; process until smooth and set aside.

2. Heat a large non-stick pot or wok over medium-high heat. Add the onions and carrots and one tablespoon of water, cover, and cook until softened,

stirring often and adding more water as necessary to prevent burning—about 5 minutes.

3. Add the spice paste from the blender and cook, stirring, for 2 minutes. Add the cauliflower and kidney beans. Cover and turn heat to low.

4. Put the tomato paste and 1 ¼ cup water in the blender and blend thoroughly. Add the tomato paste mixture to the vegetables, cover, and cook for 5 minutes. Add the zucchini and bell pepper, season with pepper and salt (if using), and continue cooking, covered, until the vegetables are tender, but not mushy, about 5 -10 minutes.

5. Add the peas and allow to heat through for a couple of minutes. Serve alone or over basmati rice or other grain.

4. Stews And Soups

Lemon Lentil Rosemary Soup

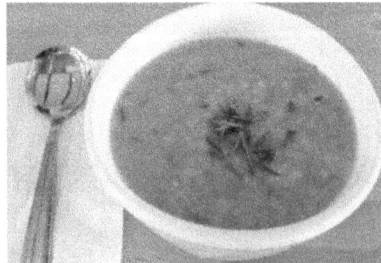

Serves: 4

Cook Time: 6 hours
Ingredients

- 6 carrots diced
- 1 large onion diced
- 4 cloves garlic minced
- 1 yellow pepper chopped
- ⅛ teaspoon cayenne pepper
- 3 cups red lentils
- 4 cups chicken broth
- 2-¾ cups water
- 1-½ teaspoons salt
- 1 lemon zest and juice
- 1 tablespoon fresh rosemary chopped

Directions

1. In a six quart slow cooker, add all ingredients EXCEPT lemon zest and juice and rosemary.
2. Cook on LOW for 6 hours.
3. Stir in lemon zest, juice and rosemary.
4. Season with additional salt and pepper to taste.
5. Ladle into bowls and garnish with additional chopped rosemary if desired.

Navy Bean Soup

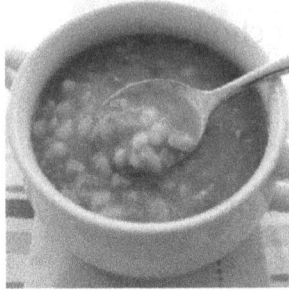

Serves: 4

Cook Time: 5 hours
Ingredients

- 4 tbsp olive oil

- 1 medium onion, chopped

- 3 cloves garlic, minced

- 5 carrots, chopped

- 5 stalks of celery, chopped

- 1lb dry navy beans, washed and checked (do not use kidney or cannellini beans)

- 1 bay leaf

- 1 tsp dried rosemary

- ½ tsp dried thyme

- ½ tsp paprika

- 4 cups chicken or vegetable stock

- 3 cups water
- Pepper to taste
- OPTIONAL - add crumbled bacon or leftover ham (cubed)

Directions

1. Combine all of the above ingredients into the slow cooker and stir.
2. Set to cook on high for 4-5 hours or low for 8 hours
3. Once cooked, add salt and slightly mash up some of the beans against the side of the slow cooker to thicken the soup.
4. Serve with some crusty bread and salty hard cheese and enjoy!

Chard, Lentil & Potato Slow Cooker Soup

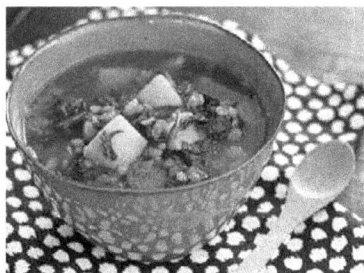

-=Serves: 4

Cook Time: 8 hours
Ingredients

- 1 tbsp. olive oil
- 1 large yellow onion, chopped
- 1 celery stalk, sliced
- 1 large carrot, sliced
- 2 garlic cloves, minced
- 1 large bunch Swiss chard, leaves torn into bite-sized pieces and stems sliced
- 1 c. dried brown lentils, picked over and rinsed
- 4 medium Yukon Gold potatoes, cut into 1-inch pieces
- 6 c. vegetable broth
- 1 tbsp. soy sauce or tamari
- salt and pepper to taste

Directions

1. Heat oil in a large skillet over medium heat. Add onion, celery, carrot, garlic, and stems from Swiss chard. Cover and cook until softened, about 8-10 minutes, stirring occasionally.

2. Add cooked vegetable mixture, lentils, potatoes, broth, and soy sauce in a 4- to 6-quart slow cooker. Stir to combine, cover, and cook on low heat for 8 hours.

3. Just before soup is finished cooking, bring a large pot of water to a boil. Place reserved chard leaves in boiling water and cook until tender, about 5

minutes. Drain well and stir into soup. Season with salt and pepper to taste.

Vegan Lasagna Soup

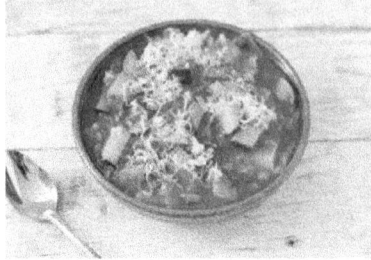

Serves: 4

Cook Time: 3 hours
Ingredients

For the Lasagna Soup

- 4 ½ cups vegetable broth
- 1 medium onion diced
- 3 garlic cloves minced
- ¾ cup dried brown lentils
- 1 teaspoon dried basil
- 1 teaspoon dried oregano
- 1 14 ounce can diced tomatoes
- 1 14 ounce can crushed tomatoes
- 8 lasagna noodles broken into pieces
- 3 cups chopped spinach leaves

For the Vegan Pesto Ricotta

- 1 cup raw cashews soaked in water 4 to 8 hours, drained and rinsed
- ¼ cup unflavored soy or almond milk
- ¼ pound extra firm tofu drained
- 3 to 4 tablespoons prepared vegan pesto to taste
- 1 tablespoon lemon juice
- salt and pepper to taste

Directions

1. Make the Lasagna Soup

2. Place broth, onion, garlic, basil, oregano and lentils into slow cooker and stir a few times to blend. Set the slow cooker to high and cover. Allow to cook until lentils are just a bit on the firm side, about 2 hours.

3. Add diced and crushed tomatoes to the slow cooker and stir. Allow to continue cooking on high for 2 to 3 hours more.

4. Add noodles and spinach to the slow cooker and give the mixture a stir. Allow to cook until noodles are tender and spinach is wilted, about 12 minutes.

5. Season the soup with salt and pepper to taste.

6. Make the Vegan Pesto Ricotta

7. Place cashews, and milk into food processor and blend until smooth. Add tofu and pulse a few times, just until the mixture takes on a ricotta-like texture. Add pesto to taste, lemon juice, and season with salt and pepper to taste.

Vegan Coconut Curry Chickpea Lentil Soup

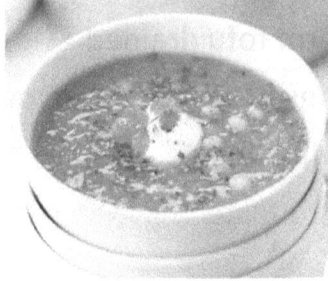

Serves: 4

Cook Time: 4 hours
Ingredients

- 2 (15 ounce) cans chickpeas (garbanzo beans), drained and rinsed
- 1 cup dry lentils, picked over and rinsed
- 1 large sweet potato, cut into small cubes
- 1 (15 ounce) can lite coconut milk
- 2 tablespoons curry powder (I used mild curry)
- 1 teaspoon ground turmeric
- 1 teaspoon ground ginger
- ½ teaspoon salt
- ¼ teaspoon pepper
- 6 cups vegetable broth

Directions

1. Put all ingredients in the slow cooker and mix well. Cook on high heat for 4 hours. (I have not tried it, but cooking it on low heat for 8 hours would most likely work also.)
2. Taste and add more salt and pepper if you prefer. Enjoy!

Slow-Cooker Hot And Sour Soup

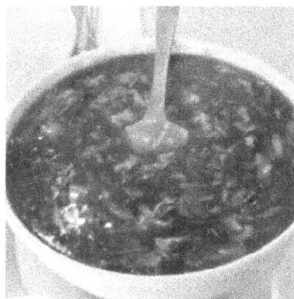

Serves: 4

Cook Time: 6 hours
Ingredients

- 1 10-ounce package sliced mushrooms (280g)
- 8 fresh shiitake mushrooms , stems removed and caps sliced
- 1 8-ounce can bamboo shoots, drained and jullienned (225g)
- 4 cloves garlic , minced

- 1 15-ounce package firm or silken tofu, cubed (420g)
- 2 tablespoons grated fresh ginger, divided (16g)
- 4 cups water (940ml)
- 2 tablespoons vegan chicken-flavored bouillon (16g)
- 2 tablespoons soy sauce (or tamari, for gluten-free) (30ml)
- 1 teaspoon sesame oil , plus extra for drizzling (Susan's note: I didn't need the extra)
- 1 teaspoon chili paste
- 2 tablespoons rice wine vinegar or apple cider vinegar (30ml)
- 1 ½ cups fresh or frozen peas (225g)

Directions

1. The Night Before: Store the cut-up mushrooms, bamboo shoots, garlic, and tofu in an airtight container in the fridge. Store the prepared ginger in another airtight container in the fridge.

2. In the Morning: Combine the mushrooms, bamboo, shoots, garlic, tofu, 1 tablespoon (8g) of the ginger, water, bouillon, soy sauce, sesame oil, chili paste, and vinegar in the slow cooker. Cook on low for 8 hours.

3. A few minutes before serving, add the peas and the remaining 1 tablespoon (8g) ginger and stir to combine. Taste the broth and add more vinegar or chili if needed. Drizzle a few drops of sesame oil on

top of each serving. If you like it milder and your friends like it hot, serve the chili paste on the side.

Vegan Sweet Potato Soup

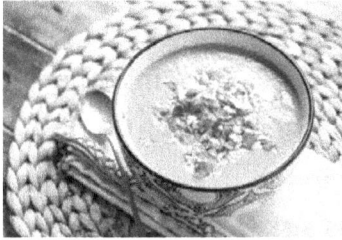

Serves: 4

Cook Time: 5 hours
Ingredients

- 5 cups low sodium vegetable broth
- 3 large sweet potatoes peeled and chopped
- 1 cup onion chopped
- 2 stalks celery chopped
- 2 cloves garlic crushed
- 1 cup plant milk (I use rice milk)
- 1 tsp. dried tarragon
- 1 tsp. McCormick Pinch Perfect Salt Free Seasoning
- 2 cups baby spinach
- 6-8 Tbsp. sliced almonds
- sea salt and ground black pepper to taste

Directions

1. Add broth, sweet potatoes, onion, celery, and garlic to a 4-quart slow cooker.
2. Cook on low for 8 hours or high for 5 hours (or until potatoes are soft). *
3. Turn off slow cooker and add plant milk, tarragon and Pinch Perfect Seasoning and blend 1-2 minutes with an immersion blender until soup is smooth. **
4. Stir in baby spinach, cover and let sit for 20 minutes until spinach is soft.
5. Ladle into soup bowls.
6. Sprinkle each bowl with 1 tbs sliced almonds, sea salt and ground black pepper to taste.

Tomato-Basil Tortellini Soup

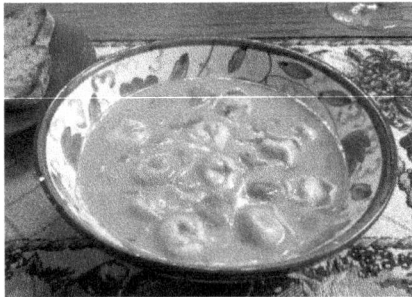

Serves: 4

Cook Time: 6 hours
Ingredients

- 1 ¾ cup diced carrots (3 medium)

- 1 ¾ cup diced yellow onion (1 large)
- 2 Tbsp olive oil
- 5 cloves garlic , minced
- 3 (28 oz) cans whole Roma tomatoes
- 1 (32 oz) carton vegetable broth
- ⅓ cup chopped fresh basil , plus more for garnish
- 2 bay leaves
- 1 Tbsp granulated sugar
- Salt and freshly ground black pepper , to taste
- 16 oz refrigerated three cheese tortellini
- ¾ cup heavy cream
- Parmesan , shredded, for serving

Directions

1. Heat olive oil in a large skillet over medium-high heat. Add carrots and onion and saute 3 - 4 minutes, add garlic and saute 1 minute longer. Pour mixture into a 6 or 7 quart slow cooker along with tomatoes, vegetable broth, basil, bay leaves, sugar. Stir and season with salt and pepper to taste. Cover slow cooker and cook on LOW 6 - 7 hours or HIGH 3 - 3 ½ hours.

2. Remove bay leaves then puree mixture well with an emulsion blender (or carefully in small batches in a blender. If your slow cooker doesn't keep all the moisture in well while cooking, you may need to add in ½ cup water or so at this point so the soup

isn't too thick). Stir in tortellini, cover and cook on HIGH heat 15 minutes longer (or until heated through). Reduce heat to warm, stir in heavy cream. Serve topped with parmesan cheese and fresh basil.

Vegetable Soup

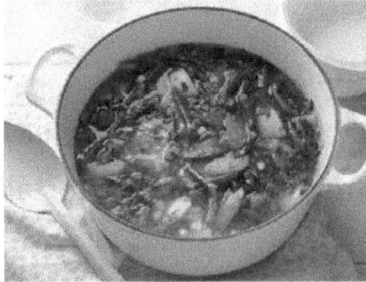

Serves: 4

Cook Time: 8 hours
Ingredients

- 4 cups vegetable broth
- 4 cups tomato juice
- 1 cup sliced carrots
- 1 cup sliced celery
- ½ cup chopped onion
- 1 cup sliced mushrooms
- 1 can of diced tomatoes
- 1 tablespoon dried basil
- 1 teaspoon salt

- ¼ teaspoon pepper
- 2 cups uncooked rotini pasta
- shredded Parmesan cheese for topping if desired

Directions

1. Add all the ingredients except the uncooked pasta and cheese to a 6 quart crock pot.
2. Cover and cook on low heat for 8 hours.
3. Add pasta and stir. Turn heat setting to high and cook for 20-30 minutes or until pasta is done.
4. Serve with each bowl topped with a sprinkling of cheese.

Thai-Inspired Butternut Squash Soup

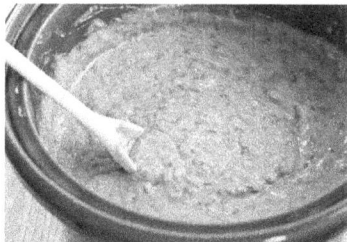

Serves: 4

Cook Time: 3 hours

Ingredients

- 2 lbs. peeled and cubed butternut squash
- 1 cup vegetable stock (vegetable broth in a can is fine)
- salt and fresh ground black pepper to taste
- 2 tsp. olive oil
- 1 onion, finely chopped
- 2 tsp. minced garlic (minced garlic from a jar is fine)
- 1 tsp. minced ginger root (pureed ginger from a jar is fine)
- 1 red bell pepper, seeds removed and finely chopped
- 1 can (14 oz.) light Thai Coconut Milk
- 2 T Thai Red Curry Paste
- ½ cup natural peanut butter (without added sugar)
- 1 T brown sugar, Stevia in the Raw granulated sweetener, or Splenda (use Stevia or Splenda for South Beach Diet)
- 2 tsp. Fish Sauce (use vegan "fish sauce" for vegan version, or replace with soy sauce if you're not a fan of fish sauce)
- 2 T fresh-squeezed lime juice
- ⅓ cup finely chopped cilantro
- extra chopped cilantro and chopped peanuts for serving (optional)
- Sriracha Rooster Sauce for serving (optional)

Directions

1. Peel the butternut squash and cut into cubes if you're starting with a whole squash. (Here's How to Peel and Cut Up a Butternut Squash if you haven't done it.) Put the squash cubes and vegetable stock into the slow cooker, season squash generously with salt and fresh-ground black pepper, and cook on high for 2 hours, or until the squash is soft enough to mash easily. When it's soft, use a food processor, blender, or Immersion Blender to puree the squash, being careful with the hot food.

2. Heat the oil in a large non-stick frying pan, add onion and saute until well-browned, about 8 minutes. Add the minced garlic, minced ginger, and diced red bell pepper and saute about a minute more. Then add the coconut milk, Thai Red Curry Paste, and peanut butter and heat just until the curry paste and peanut butter is melted into the coconut milk. Add the sweetener and fish sauce.

3. Stir the coconut milk mixture into the pureed squash, turn slow cooker to low and cook for 1 hour more. Stir in the chopped cilantro and fresh lime juice and cook about 15 minutes more. Serve hot, garnished with more chopped cilantro and chopped peanuts if desired. If you'd like more heat, shake in a little Sriracha Sauce.

Loaded Baked Potato Soup

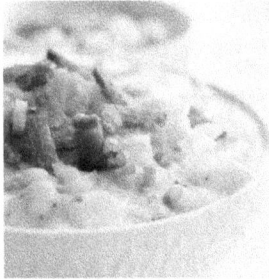

Serves: 4

Cook Time: 4 hours
Ingredients

- 5 medium/standard-sized russet potatoes, peeled and chopped into ½-inch cubes
- ½ cup finely diced celery (approximately 3 stalks)
- 1 onion, diced
- 3 cups of vegetable broth
- 3 cloves of garlic, minced
- ¼ cup salted butter
- ½ cup parmesan cheese, grated
- ½ cup sharp cheddar, grated
- a few cranks of ground black pepper
- 1 tsp kosher salt
- ¼ tsp garlic powder
- ¼ tsp red pepper flakes

154

- ½ tsp dried dill (add ¼ tsp first, taste, then double if you love it!)
- TASTY TOPPINGS:
- plain greek yogurt or sour cream
- freshly grated cheddar cheese
- zesty red pepper flakes
- chopped green onion

Directions

1. Chop your veggies and toss em in the pot!
2. Next add veggie broth, garlic, butter, salt, and pepper.
3. Set your slow cooker to HIGH and cook for 4 hours, or, if you›re gone for the day, set it to LOW for 8 hours.
4. After returning to your slow cooker, you have a very important (ok not that important) decision to make. Do you want your soup chunky or smooth?
5. For smooth soup, use a potato masher or even an immersion blender to creamify the soup.
6. For chunky potato soup, grab a wooden spoon and mash the potatoes partially. I went the fabulously chunky route and it came out deliciously thick and hearty.
7. Ready to eat? Simply mix in your cheese, spices, and a spoonful or two of green onions. Taste, season as needed, toss on some toppings, and dig in! I wound up adding extra dill and a little more garlic powder...

The flavor was spot on and I didn't miss bacon one bit! Success!

Asian Corn Cabbage Soup

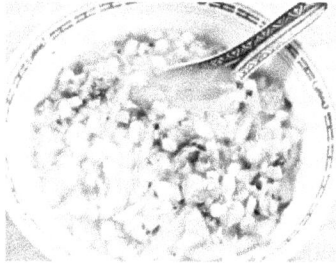

Serves: 4

Cook Time: 7 hours
Ingredients

- ½ small onion, minced
- 1 tablespoon (15 ml) olive oil (*or sauté in water)
- 2 cloves garlic, minced
- 1 ½ cups (105 g) minced mushrooms
- Pinch of salt
- 2 to 3 teaspoons (10-15 g) minced ginger
- 4 cups (356 g) chopped cabbage
- 2 cups (282 g) corn kernels (frozen or fresh)
- 4 cups (946 ml) water
- 1 tablespoon (5 g) nutritional yeast
- 2 teaspoons (10 ml) vegetable bouillon
- 1 teaspoon sesame oil

- ½ to 1 teaspoon sriracha sauce
- 1 teaspoon light soy sauce

Directions

1. To prep the night before, sauté the onion in oil (or water) until it's translucent, then add the garlic and cook one more minute. Add mushrooms and a pinch of salt. Sauté until the mushrooms have cooked down and released their liquid. Store the cooked mixture with cut cabbage and corn in the refrigerator overnight.

2. In the morning, add everything except sesame, sriracha and soy sauce (or coconut aminos) to your 4-quart (4-L) slow cooker. Cook 7 to 9 hours on low.

3. Before serving, add sesame, sriracha and soy sauce (or coconut aminos). Adjust seasonings if needed.

Creole Corn And Okra Soup

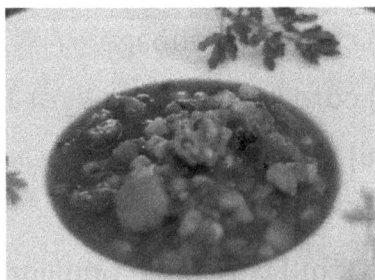

Serves: 4

Cook Time: 7 hours
Ingredients

- 2 tablespoons olive oil (or use broth to make oil-free)
- ½ medium onion, minced
- ½ medium green pepper, minced
- 3 cloves garlic, minced
- 3 cups vegetable broth (or water with 2 veggie bouillon cubes)
- 1 (16 oz/454 g) bag frozen sliced okra
- 2 cups (11 oz/ 328 g) frozen corn kernels
- 1 (28 oz/794 g) can of crushed tomatoes (fire roasted or plain)
- 1 ½ teaspoon smoked paprika (or plain paprika plus a few drops of liquid smoke)
- 1 teaspoon thyme
- 1 teaspoon oregano
- 1 teaspoon marjoram
- ¼ to ½ teaspoon of ground cayenne pepper (depending on your love of heat)
- salt and pepper, to taste

Directions

1. Heat oil over medium heat and add in the onion once it's hot.

2. Sauté until the onions become translucent, about 5 minutes.

3. Add green pepper and garlic then sauté 3 minutes more.

4. Stir in the broth, okra, corn, tomatoes and all spices except for the salt and pepper.

5. Simmer for 20 to 30 minutes over medium heat until the corn and okra are tender.

6. Before serving add salt and pepper to taste.

7. Slow cooker variation:

8. Heat oil over medium heat and add in the onion once it's hot.

9. Sauté until the onions become translucent, about 5 minutes.

10. Add the sautéed onions and everything else except the salt and black pepper and cook on low for 7 to 10 hours.

11. Before serving add salt and pepper to taste.

Slow-Cooked Minestrone Soup

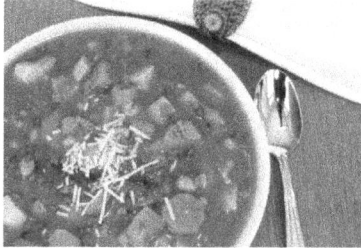

Serves: 4

Cook Time: 6 hours
Ingredients

- 4 cups vegetable broth
- 4 cups diced tomatoes
- 1 tbsp. chopped fresh basil
- ½ tsp. oregano
- 3 carrots, chopped
- 3 stalks celery, chopped
- ½ onion, chopped
- 2 zucchinis, chopped
- 2 yellow crookneck squash, chopped
- 1 cup green beans, chopped
- 3 cloves garlic, minced
- 2 bay leaves
- Salt and pepper to taste

- 1 ½ cups macaroni pasta

Directions

1. Combine all ingredients except pasta in a crock pot. Cook on low for 6-8 hours.
2. Add the pasta and cook on high for 20-30 minutes, or until pasta is done cooking.
3. Remove bay leaves before serving.

Teriyaki Mushrooms

Ingredients:

5-6 cups small mushrooms, stems removed

2 cups teriyaki sauce

2 cups water

2 TBSP olive oil

1 cup raw honey

½ tsp pepper

¼ tsp ginger

Directions:

Place mushrooms in the slow cooker and put remaining ingredients on top. Stir to combine. Cover and cook on low for 6 hours, stirring occasionally.

Pumpkin Pie Dip

Ingredients:

2 cups pumpkin puree

1 cup cashew cream

2 TBSP almond butter

2 tsp pumpkin pie spice

1 tsp vanilla extract

¼ cup honey

Directions:

Combine all ingredients in your slow cooker and stir until completely mixed. Cover and cook on low for 1-2 hours. Serve with gingersnaps or apple slices.

Sweet and Sour Tofu

Ingredients:

1 lb extra firm tofu

2 TBSP canola oil

1 TBSP cornstarch

½ yellow onion, chopped

1 yellow bell pepper

1 cup broccoli florets

1 cup carrots, sliced

1 cup sliced water chestnuts

10 oz. sweet and sour sauce

Directions:

Press moisture out of the tofu and cut into bite size cubes. Coat the cubes with cornstarch and then fry in a canola oil for about 15 minutes or until crunchy on the outside. Place tofu and vegetables in your slow cooker and cover with sweet and sour sauce. Stir together and cover. Cook on low for 3 hours.

Sweet and Spicy Pecans

Ingredients:

1/4 cup coconut oil

6 cups pecans

2 tsp chili powder

2 tsp sugar

½ tsp cinnamon

Directions:

Heat the coconut oil in your slow cooker on high for 15 minutes or until melted. Pour in the pecans and stir until they are coated in the melted oil. Cover and cook on high for two hours. Then take the lid off the slow cooker and continue cooking on high for 2 ½ more hours, stirring every half hour. Sprinkle seasonings on top and spread on a baking sheet to cool.

Eggplant Hummus

Ingredients:

1 eggplant

2 garlic cloves

Juice from 1 lemon

2 TBSP sesame paste

1 TBSP dried parsley

Salt and pepper to taste

Directions:

Wash the eggplant and poke with a fork 4-5 times. Place it in the slow cooker and cover. Cover on high for 3 hours. Using tongs, remove the eggplant and cut it in half. Scrape out the seeds and discard. Now use a spoon to scoop out the flesh and place it in your blender with remaining ingredients. Puree until smooth.

Wasabi Almonds

Ingredients:

1 pound raw almonds

1 TBSP water

1 TBSP soy sauce

2 TBSP coconut oil, melted

2 TBSP wasabi powder

1 tsp salt

Directions:

Whisk together melted coconut oil, water, and soy sauce in a bowl. Pour in the almonds and toss to combine. Pour the almonds in a large zip-top bag and add in seasonings. Shake it to coat the almonds evenly. Now pour the almonds into your slow cooker and cover. Cover on low for 2-4 hours or until the almonds are toasted and lightly browned. Spread the almonds on a baking sheet and allow them to dry.

Creamy Vegetable Dip

Ingredients:

1/4 head of cauliflower

2 TBSP sesame paste

½ clove garlic

Juice from ½ lemon

1/8 cup water

1 TBSP olive oil

½ tomato, diced

Salt and pepper to taste

1 cup vegetable broth

Directions:

Place cauliflower and vegetable broth in slow cooker and cook on low for 4 hours. Then place cauliflower in your food processor with remaining ingredients and pulse until smooth.

Southern Boiled Peanuts

Ingredients:

2 pounds raw peanuts, in shell

¾ cup salt

12 cups water

Directions:

Combine all ingredients in the slow cooker and cover. Cook on high for 18 hours or until peanuts are soft. Drain and serve warm or store in refrigerator.

Vegan Chili Con Queso

Ingredients:

16 oz. cashew cream or other cream cheese substitute

4 cups meatless chili

½ cup chopped green chilies

1 jar of salsa

1 red onion, minced

Directions:

Combine all ingredients in the slow cooker and cover. Cook on high for one hour. Stir well before serving.

Slow Cooker Salsa

Ingredients:

10 tomatoes, cored and chopped

2 garlic cloves, minced

1 onion, chopped

2 jalapeno peppers, chopped

½ tsp Salt

½ tsp cayenne pepper

¼ cup cilantro leaves, chopped

Directions:

Combine all ingredients except cilantro in slow cooker. Cover and cook on high for 1 hour or until you reach desired consistency. Stir in cilantro and serve with tortilla chips.

Rosemary Olive Oil Bread

Ingredients:

3 ½ cups all purpose flour

1 packet dry active yeast

1 ¼ cups warm water

¼ cup fresh rosemary, chopped, divided

3 TBSP olive oil

1 tsp sugar

1 tsp sea salt, divided

Directions:

In a large bowl, combine water, yeast, and sugar. Allow it sit and proof for 10 minutes. It will look foamy when it's ready. Stir in ½ tsp Salt, ½ of rosemary, 3 TBSP olive oil, and all of the flour. Mix until completely combined. Use your hands to form the dough if necessary.

Grease a large bowl and place dough inside. Cover with a kitchen towel and leave in a warm area for one hour to rise. Remove the dough and roll into a ball. Allow it sit for another 20 minutes for the second rise.

Turn your slow cooker on high and line it with two pieces of parchment paper, allowing a few inches to hang out on the sides of the slow cooker. Lay dough inside the slow cooker and sprinkle with salt and remaining rosemary.

Cover and cook for two hours. Then lift it out of the slow cooker and allow to cool. For a crunchier crust, place under the broiler for around 3 minutes.

Pumpkin Bread

Ingredients:

1 can of pumpkin puree (15 oz)

½ cup vegetable oil

½ cup sugar

½ cup packed brown sugar

1 ½ cups flour

¼ tsp Salt

1 tsp pumpkin pie spice

1 tsp baking soda

1 banana, pureed

Directions:

In a large bowl, beat together oil, sugar, and brown sugar. Stir in the pureed banana and pumpkin. Add remaining ingredients and mix to combine. Pour batter into a well greased bread pan. Add two cups of water to the slow cooker and lay the pan inside. Cover the top of the slow cooker with 8-10 paper towels to keep condensation from dripping down onto the bread. Place the lid on top and cook on high for 2 ½ to 3 hours or until a toothpick comes out clean.

Chocolate Chip Zucchini Bread

Ingredients:

1 cup applesauce

1 ½ cups sugar

3 cups flour

1 tsp baking soda

½ tsp baking powder

2 tsp cinnamon

3 tsp vanilla

¼ tsp Salt

2 cups peeled and grated zucchini

1 cup Vegan chocolate chips

1 ½ bananas, pureed (or other substitute for 3 eggs)

Directions:

Spray a 3-qt. slow cooker with non-stick spray. In a large mixing bowl, combine pureed banana, sugar, and applesauce. Next, stir in flour, baking powder, baking soda, cinnamon, Salt, and vanilla. Last, mix in zucchini and fold in chocolate chips. Pour batter into the slow cooker. Cook on low for 2-3 hours or until toothpick comes out clean. Flip onto a plate and allow to cool before slicing.

Apple Bread

Ingredients:

1 ½ cups Bisquick or other baking mix

½ cup coconut milk

1 cup apple pie filling

¼ cup vegetable oil

Directions:

Mix together bisquick, coconut milk, and oil. Stir in apple pie filling and then pour batter into your greased slow cooker. Cook on high for 1 hour to 1 ½ hours. It's done when a toothpick inserted in the center comes out clean.

Apricot Nut Bread

Ingredients:

1 cup all purpose flour

½ cup whole wheat flour

2 tsp baking powder

¼ tsp baking soda

½ tsp Salt

½ cup sugar

¾ cup almond milk

¼ cup vegetable oil
¾ cup dried apricots, chopped

1 TBSP grated orange peel

1 cup walnuts, chopped

Directions:

Combine dry ingredients in a large bowl. Add in almond milk, oil, and orange peel. Stir to combine. Fold in apricots and walnuts and pour into a well greased bread pan. Place on a rack in the slow cooker and cover, leaving a little room for steam to escape. Cook on high for 4-6 hours.

Slow Cooker Amish White Bread

Ingredients:

1 packet fast acting yeast

2 TBSP sugar

½ tsp Salt

1 ½ cups flour

½ cup hot water (not boiling)

1 TBSP oil

Directions:
Combine yeast, sugar, Salt, and flour in a large bowl, Slowly add in water and oil until dough forms. Form into a bowl and place in a greased bowl. Cover with a towel and allow to rise in a warm place for 1 hour or until doubled in size. Line slow cooker with parchment paper and place dough inside. Cover and cook on low for 1 ½ to 2 hours.

Whole Wheat Bread

Ingredients:

1 TBSP yeast

¼ cup warm water

1 cup warm almond milk

¼ cup rolled oats

1 tsp Salt

2 TBSP olive oil

2 TBSP raw honey

½ banana, mashed

¼ cup milet

2 TBSP ground flax seed

2 ¾ cup whole wheat flour

Directions:

In a large bowl, dissolve yeast in warm water and allow to proof for 10 minutes. It is done when it is bubbly and foamy on top. Add in remaining ingredients to form a dough and then knead for 5 minutes, until smooth and elastic. Place prepared dough into a greased bread pan. Add 1 cup water to your slow cooker and place bread pan on top. Cover and bake on high for 3 hours. Crack slow cooker to allow steam to vent if you notice condensation collecting on top.

Orange Cranberry Bread

Ingredients:

1 cup all purpose flour

½ cup whole wheat flour

2 tsp baking powder

¼ tsp baking soda

½ tsp Salt

½ cup sugar

¾ cup almond milk

¼ cup vegetable oil
¾ cup dried cranberries, chopped

2 TBSP grated orange peel

1 cup walnuts, chopped

Directions:

Combine dry ingredients in a large bowl. Add in almond milk, oil, and orange peel. Stir to combine. Fold in cranberries and walnuts and pour into a well greased bread pan. Place on a rack in the slow cooker and cover, leaving a little room for steam to escape. Cook on high for 4-6 hours.

Breakfast Risotto

Ingredients:

3 gala apples, chopped

1 ½ tsp cinnamon

1/8 tsp nutmeg

1/8 tsp cloves

¼ tsp Salt

¼ cup coconut oil

1/3 cup brown sugar

1 ½ cups Arborio rice

3 cups apple juice

1 cup almond milk

Directions:

Turn your crock to high and add the coconut oil so it can start melting. Chop apples while you wait. Stir in the rice to the coconut oil, then add apples and remaining ingredients. Cover and cook on high for 5 hours or low for 6-7 hours.

Cranberry Fig Oatmeal

Ingredients:

1 cup steel cut oats

1 cup dried cranberries

1 cup dried figs

4 cups water

1/2 cup almond milk

Directions:

Combine all ingredients in the slow cooker and stir to combine. Cover and cook on low for 8 to 9 hours.

Apple Walnut Oatmeal

Ingredients:

1 cup steel cut oats

1 cup chopped apples

1 cup chopped walnuts

4 cups water

1/2 cup almond milk

Directions:

Combine all ingredients in the slow cooker and stir to combine. Cover and cook on low for 8 to 9 hours.

Peaches and Cream Breakfast Cereal

Ingredients:

1 1/4 cups steel cut oats

1 can peaches, diced

1 cup chopped walnuts

4 cups water

1 cup coconut milk

Directions:

Combine all ingredients in the slow cooker and stir to combine. Cover and cook on low for 8 to 9 hours.

Cinnamon Applesauce

Ingredients:

3 1/2 lbs granny smith apples, peeled, cored, and sliced

1/2 cup packed brown sugar

1 1/2 TBSP fresh lemon juice

1/4 tsp ground cinnamon

Directions:

Combine all ingredients in the slow cooker and cook on high for 3 hours or on low for 5-6 hours. Mash with a potato masher and serve warm.

Pumpkin Spice Steel Cut Oats

Ingredients:

1 1/2 cup steel cut oats

4 cups water

1/8 cup pumpkin puree

1 tsp pumpkin pie spice

1 TBSP brown sugar

1 TBSP sugar

Directions:

Combine all ingredients in the slow cooker and stir to combine. Cover and cook on low for 8-9 hours.

Morning Plum Pudding

Ingredients:

2 cups dried, pitted plums

water to cover prunes

2/3 cup boiling water

1 cup raw honey

Zest from ½ orange

¼ cup almonds, chopped

Directions:

Soak the plums in water overnight. Take them out of the water and put in slow cooker. Add in 2/3 cup boiling water, honey, and orange zest. Cover and cook on high for 3 hours. Pour the plum pudding in a serving dish and chill for at least 2 hours. Top with chopped almonds and serve.

Warm Spiced Fruit

Ingredients:

3 cups sliced peaches

1 can pineapple tidbits with liquid

3 cups pear slices

½ cup green seedless grapes, halved

½ cup maraschino cherries, halved

1 ½ tsp cinnamon

1 tsp nutmeg

½ cup honey

4 TBSP coconut oil

½ cup coconut milk

Directions:

Combine all ingredients in the slow cooker and cover. Cook on low for 4-6 hours. Serve with whipped coconut cream if desired.

Vegan Breakfast Casserole

Ingredients:

5 cups frozen hash browns

2 cups cheese substitute

1 1/2 cups almond milk

½ cup chives

1 cup frozen peas

1 tsp Salt

1 tsp pepper

1 tsp paprika

Directions:

Combine all ingredients in the slow cooker. Cover and cook on low for 6-8 hours.

Banana Bread Quinoa

Ingredients:

1 cup of quinoa

1 cup almond milk

1 tsp vanilla extract

1 cup water

1 1/2 banana (past ripe), mashed

2 tablespoons chopped walnuts

3 tablespoons brown sugar

1 1/2 tablespoons coconut oil, melted

Directions:

In a small bowl, mix the brown sugar and walnuts together. Pour quinoa, almond milk, water, butter and vanilla into the crock pot. Add the mashed banana and stir to evenly distribute. Sprinkle the sugar and walnut mixture into the quinoa and stir to combine. Cover and cook on low for 4-6 hours. Add additional almond milk as needed and add sugar to taste.

Breakfast Burrito Filling

Ingredients:

1 15oz can black beans, drained and rinsed

1 10oz can diced tomatoes with green chiles, don't drain

1 cup uncooked pearl barley

2 cups vegetable broth

¾ cups frozen corn

¼ cup chives

Juice from 1 lime

1 tsp ground cumin

1 tsp chili powder

½ tsp red pepper flakes

3 garlic cloves, minced

Directions:

Combine all ingredients in the slow cooker and cook on low for 5-6 hours. Place the filling inside warm tortillas for an instant breakfast burrito.

Baked Stuffed Apples

Ingredients:

6 large green apples

¼ cup raisins

¼ cup honey

1 tsp cinnamon

6 TBSP coconut oil

Directions:

Core apples, but leave about half an inch at the bottom. Divide raisins, honey, cinnamon, and coconut oil between the apples, stuffing the cavity where apples were cored. Placed stuffed apples in the slow cooker with ½ inch of water. Cook on low overnight.

Cherry Almond Granola

Ingredients:

5 cups old fashioned rolled oats

1 cup whole almonds

1/2 cup dried cherries

1/2 cup pepitas

1/4 cup shredded coconut

1/4 cup canola oil

1/4 cup honey

1 tsp vanilla

Directions:

Add the oats, honey, oil, almonds, and vanilla to the slow cover. Cook uncovered on high for one hour, stirring every 20 minutes. Reduce heat to low and add coconut, pepitas, and cherries. Cook on low uncovered for 4 more hours, stirring every half hour. Cook on baking sheets.

9 781990 334337